THE ULTIMATE
BODYBUILDING
COOKBOOK

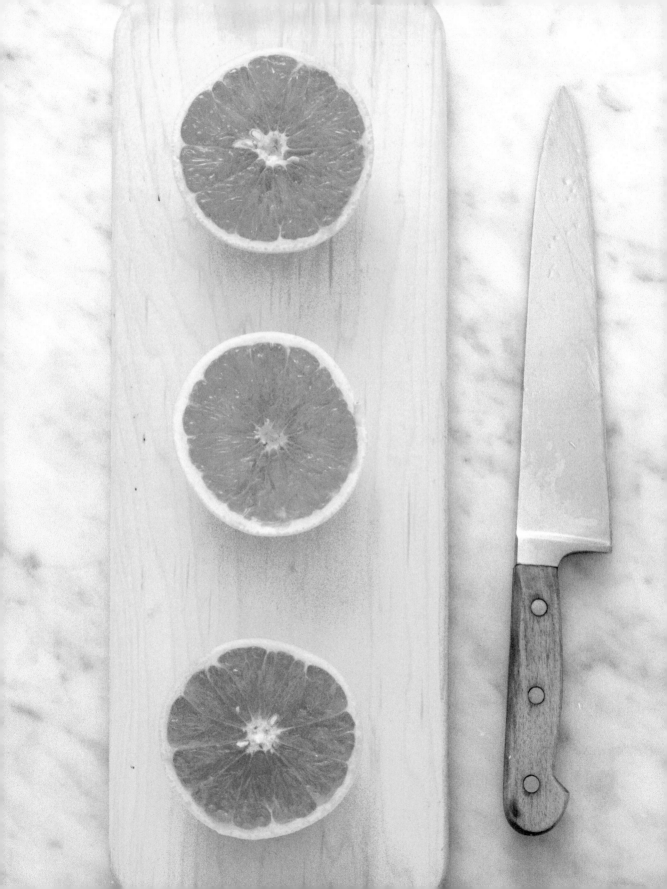

KENDALL LOU SCHMIDT

THE ULTIMATE
BODYBUILDING
COOKBOOK

High-Impact Recipes to Make
You Stronger Than Ever

ROCKRIDGE
PRESS

For general information on our other products and services or to obtain technical support, please contact our Customer Care Department within the United States at (866) 744-2665, or outside the United States at (510) 253-0500.

Rockridge Press publishes its books in a variety of electronic and print formats. Some content that appears in print may not be available in electronic books, and vice versa.

TRADEMARKS: Rockridge Press and the Rockridge Press logo are trademarks or registered trademarks of Callisto Media Inc. and/or its affiliates, in the United States and other countries, and may not be used without written permission. All other trademarks are the property of their respective owners. Rockridge Press is not associated with any product or vendor mentioned in this book.

Cover photographs: front © Paul Sirisalee/Offset

Interior photographs: © Jeff Wasserman/Stocksy p. 2, 232; © Nadine Greeff/stocksy p. 6, 66; © Kristin Duvall/stocksy p. 16, 30; © J.R. Photography/stocksy p. 108; © Andre Baranowski/StockFood p. 130; © Davide Illini/stocksy p. 146; © Harald Walker/stocksy p. 176; Adam Nixon/stocksy p 212 © Tatjana Ristanic/stocksy p. 250; author photograph © Isaac Hinds; all other photographs © shutterstock

ISBN: Print 978-1-62315-765-4 | eBook 978-1-62315-766-1

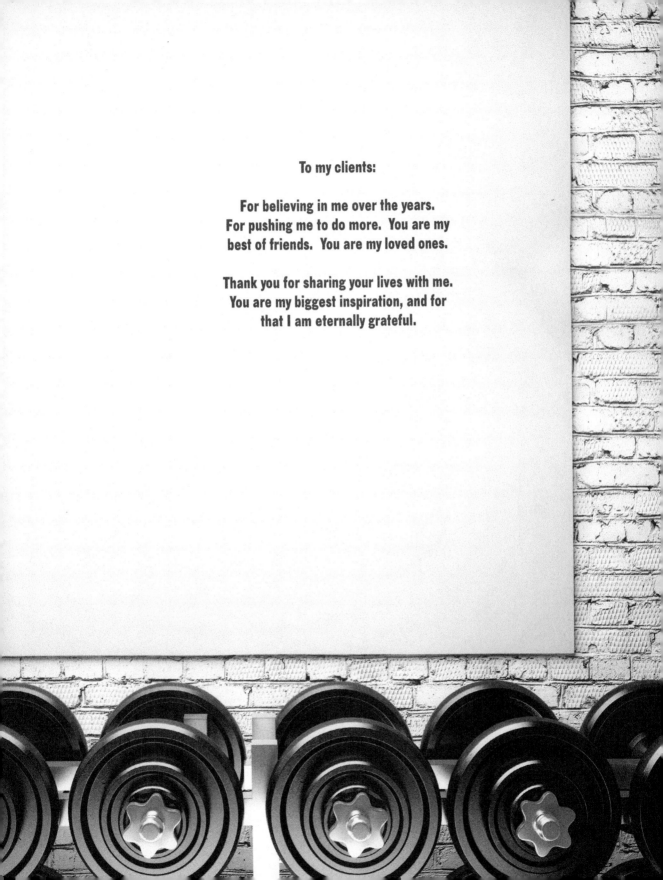

To my clients:

For believing in me over the years.
For pushing me to do more. You are my
best of friends. You are my loved ones.

Thank you for sharing your lives with me.
You are my biggest inspiration, and for
that I am eternally grateful.

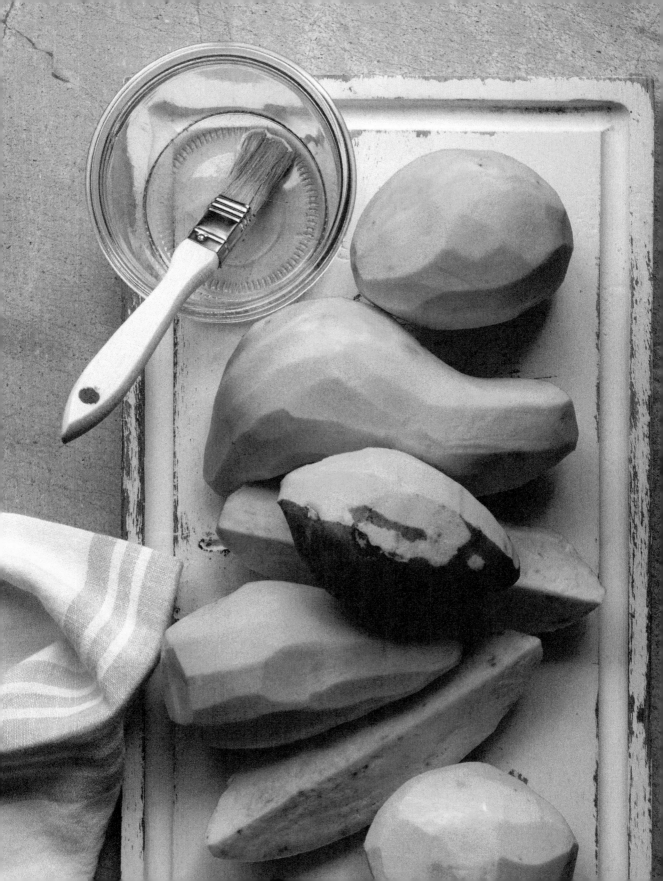

TABLE OF CONTENTS

3 BREAKFAST 41

4 CHICKEN & POULTRY

		CAL	CARB(G)	FAT (G)	PROT (G)
68	Turkey Meatballs with Marinara Sauce	117	11.9	1.3	14.4
70	Crispy Chicken with Sweet Mustard Dip	169	7	3.7	24
72	Pulled Chicken	120	3	1	22
73	Turkey Satay Skewers	100	0	1	22
74	Noodle-less Turkey Lasagna	202	20.7	1.5	31.2
76	Turkey Burger on an Eggplant Bun	149	11.1	5.6	15.5
78	Spicy Turkey Stir-Fry	175	16	1.4	24.2
79	Honey-Mushroom Chicken	168	11.3	1.8	27.3
80	Your Mom's Herb Chicken	164	0.8	6	26
81	Spicy Latin Lime Chicken	120	0	1.5	26
82	Turkey Stroganoff	174	9.5	1	33.5
83	Whole Roasted Chicken	200	1.3	12	22.7
84	Kung Pow Chicken	200	6.3	7	27.3
86	Chicken Tortilla Soup	325	39.5	3	34.8
87	Oven Roasted Turkey Breast	131	0	2.2	24.3
88	Superfood Chicken Soup	179	18.4	1.8	23.5
90	Peanut Chicken	144	3.4	2.5	28.6
92	Chicken and Veggie One-Dish Wonder	275	27.8	4	30.7
94	Grilled Lemon Chicken	141	0.5	3.9	26
96	Turkey Lettuce Wraps	100	7.5	1.5	15
98	Mandarin Chicken	231	27.5	1.5	27
100	Curry Chicken with Cauliflower "Rice"	284	20	9.8	31.8
102	Orange-Infused Chai Chicken	137	4	2	26
103	Tom Kha Gai	206	2	10	27.3
104	Roasted Garlic–Stuffed Italian Baked Chicken	172	8.1	1.5	30.8
106	Cabbage Rolls	153	7.5	1	29.4

5 BEEF 109

		CAL	CARB(G)	FAT (G)	PROT (G)
110	The Best Beef Rub	0	0	0	0
111	Grilled Marinated Steak	170	0	8.3	24
112	Garlic and Rosemary Grilled T-Bones	223	0	10.1	30.9
113	Eye Round Steak	161	0	6.3	25
114	Steak and Vegetable Soup	181	18.5	5.2	15.8
115	15-Minute Beef Chili	236	27.4	3.8	23.6
116	Sloppy Joes	193	18.4	4.8	20
117	Apples and Oats Meatloaf	235	17.5	7	26
118	Pot Roast	220	4.8	7	31
119	Slow Cooker Beef Stew	269	18.8	8.1	28.9
120	High-Heat Eye of Round Roast	185	0	5	34
121	Puerto Rican Bistec Encebollao	259	5.8	24.6	24.2
122	Salisbury Steak with Mushroom and Onion Gravy	170	3	6.9	24.9
124	Persian Beef Kebabs	152	1.2	4	25
126	Stuffed Bell Peppers	316	17.8	14.8	28.8
128	Orange Beef	245	11	12	23.25

6 PORK 131

		CAL	CARB(G)	FAT (G)	PROT (G)
132	Mexican Carnitas	205	0.5	11	26
134	Mustard-Crusted Pork Tenderloin	151	8	2.5	24
135	Asian Pork Roast	110	0	3	22
136	Pan-Seared Spicy Garlic-Ginger Pork Tenderloin	128	3.8	3.1	24
138	Almond-Crusted Pork Cutlets	295	4	19	30
139	Ham and Bean Soup	226	22.3	5.1	22.6
140	Pork and Mixed-Vegetable Stir-Fry	181	12.8	2.8	25.8
141	Pork Chile Verde	163	7.5	2.5	24.5
142	Hawaiian-Style Pork and Pineapple Skewers	179	13	2.7	24.4
144	Fennel-Crusted Roast Pork Tenderloin	120	0	2.5	23
145	Coffee-Rubbed Roast Pork Tenderloin	129	1.8	2.5	23

		CAL	CARB(G)	FAT (G)	PROT (G)
148	Garlic and Herb Shrimp	130	4	3.9	20
149	Shrimp Creole	168	11.8	3	22.3
150	Coconut Shrimp with Sweet and Spicy Dipping Sauce	168	8.7	3.5	22.2
152	Honey-Garlic Shrimp	193	17.3	4.5	20
153	Shrimp Ceviche	151	10.8	3	21
154	Cioppino	226	11.8	5.1	31.1
156	Coconut-Seared Scallops with Wilted Spinach	277	12	16	25
158	Scallop Stir-Fry	171	22	2.8	15.8
160	Maple and Mustard–Baked Scallops	125	10	1	17
161	Tuna Salad	285	7	8	48
162	Tuna Melt–Stuffed Tomatoes	189	10	4	31
163	Almond-Crusted Baked Cod	245	3	9.5	36.5
164	Salmon-Quinoa Cakes	160	14.5	5.7	13
166	Grilled Calamari Steaks with Mediterranean Topping	261	7	15	27.5
168	"Parmesan"-Crusted Tilapia	250	6	8	38
169	Crab-Stuffed Mushrooms	121	5	3.5	17.5
170	Grilled Ono with Mango-Pineapple Salsa	216	9	6.3	29.8
172	Broiled Salmon with Indian Spices	150	3	1.5	31.5
173	Grilled Balsamic and Rosemary Salmon	117	3	2	21
174	Mahimahi Tacos with Cilantro-Lime Crema	159	10.8	4.9	17.8

8 SALADS 177

	CAL	CARB(G)	FAT (G)	PROT (G)
178 Cucumber Salad	28	6.7	0	1
179 Chicken Waldorf Salad	265	17.6	9.2	29.9
180 Brussels Sprout and Berries Salad	209	23	12	3
181 Salmon Salad	174	1.2	7.5	26.3
182 Citrus-Beet Salad with Toasted Walnuts	130	23	3	4
184 Honey-Dijon Kale Salad	262	32.2	15.2	5.2
185 Spinach Caprese Salad	181	8	12	18
186 Mediterranean Bean Salad	141	18.4	6.3	6.1
187 Southwestern Salad with Pulled Chicken and Cilantro-Lime Dressing	477	26	21	51
188 Thai Peanut Salad	246	50	1	16
189 Curry Quinoa Salad	168	28.3	2.6	8.3

9 SIDES 191

	CAL	CARB(G)	FAT (G)	PROT (G)
192 Garlicky Roasted Brussels Sprouts	67.2	10.6	1	6.3
194 Zucchini Fritters	60	7.9	3.2	4.5
195 Savory Roasted Cauliflower	33	7	0	2.7
196 Protein Mashed Potatoes	132	19.8	4.5	3.8
197 Sautéed Red Cabbage with Honey and Mustard Seeds	65	11.4	1.9	1.8
198 Forbidden Fried Rice	151	25	5.5	3.6
199 Ful Medames	107	11.6	0.5	6
200 Coleslaw	50	7.7	2.2	1.4
202 Quinoa with Mushrooms and Spinach	200	32	4.6	7.8
204 Roasted Sweets and Beets	149	29.2	3	2.6
205 Chunky Apple Sauce	50	10.3	1.3	0.2
206 Stir-Fried Broccoli with Garlic	50	7.7	2.2	1.4
207 Beets and Green Beans	46	7.3	1.7	1.5
208 Sweet Potato Fries with Rosemary	125	18.2	5.4	1.4
209 Creamy Cucumber Salad	44	7	0	4.7
210 Spinach and Spaghetti Squash Soufflé	59	5.3	2.8	6.7

INTRODUCTION

In the pursuit of excellent physique, optimal performance, and our best possible self we flock to the gym. Repeatedly picking up heavy objects, climbing up stairs that lead nowhere, running in place, grunting, sweating, giving it our all. And, for what? We do it for that moment we realize that heavy feels light, the day that hard becomes easy, and goals become reality. We do it for the new vein on our bicep, the clothes we buy in a new size, the new shape we see in the mirror. We do it for the excitement it gives us, the sense of accomplishment we feel, and the trophies we take home.

You can spend a lifetime in the gym, spilling every drop of blood, sweat and tears you have, but you'll never get best results without the right diet. The food you eat is the fuel that powers your body, and the building blocks it uses to build new tissue. I'm living proof of that corollary. I've made many mistakes in my own pursuit of fitness. There is so much advice out there—a lot of it contradicting itself—that I reached many dead ends before finding my way out of the maze. On my journey here, I followed fad diets that had me cutting out healthy fats, unknowingly consumed too few carbs or too few calories, ate low-quality foods that left me feeling so deprived that each fall off the wagon would be bigger than the previous. All I ended up with was short-lived results, a damaged metabolism, and a nutrition regime that negatively affected my mood, performance, and appearance. So, what did I do? I realized that following this fad, then another one, and so on, was not helping. What my body and mind needed was good nutrition, followed consistently. Getting results is easy when you know what to do, and when you do it the right way you also get to keep them for the long term.

This book will give you all the knowledge you need to custom-build a diet that is right for you, a diet that will make you stronger, leaner, and healthier. My goal is to help and inspire everyone who reads it. Whatever your motivation, whatever your goal, whatever your gender, age, or weight, the recipes in this book can help you become your best self.

There are no fancy gadgets and ingredients. You'll find common kitchen utensils and cooking skills your mom or roommate taught you and you'll be able to tackle any of the 150 recipes in this book in a breeze. The recipes are versatile and easy. Many are designed to be prepared in bulk for your weekly meal prep, or whipped up within minutes after a long day and a hard workout. The ingredients are inexpensive, and easy to find. They have also been selected with the intention of maximizing gains, so you'll be getting the most out of every calorie you eat and out of every minute you spend in the gym. Servings are also set in portions that allow the recipes to be universal. A 300-lb bodybuilder, a 130-lb bikini competitor, a marathon runner, a CrossFit fanatic, and my 91-year-old grandma could all sit down at the same dinner table and share a meal. They wouldn't all eat the same number of servings; they wouldn't all load up their plates the same way. But, they could all eat the same recipes together, and they would all think they were delicious.

Let's be honest: The common curse of bodybuilding diets is blandness. I am here to demolish that myth. A strict fitness regime and delicious food shouldn't be mutually exclusive. You *can* have the best of both worlds, and get amazing results at the same time.

CHAPTER ONE

BODYBUILDING IS 50% NUTRITION

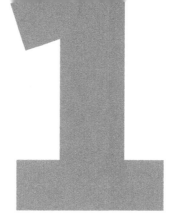

No amount of exercise can make up for a poor diet. If you're eating too much protein or not enough of it, or too few calories, you will not cut fat, you will not gain muscle. There is nothing more discouraging than not getting results, which is why most people give up.

But if you make intelligent changes to your eating habits, you can accomplish anything. Your body will begin to respond the way you want it to. It will build muscle. It will burn fat. It will get stronger and faster and more powerful. If you want all that to happen, you must give it the nutrients it needs, because a consistent fitness routine is only as good as the diet fueling it. The food you eat is more than just calories, it provides the building blocks your body uses to produce hormones, build new muscle, and perform cellular functions—all of which are necessary for achieving the best version of yourself.

The recipes in this book include ingredients proven to help build muscle and burn fat, and are backed by studies on optimal macronutrient ratios and nutrient timing, and this first chapter sets out to explain how to make this book work for you and your goals. Once you have an idea of the basic principles, you'll be able to calculate your own caloric needs. From there it is easy to pick out recipes with the right amount of protein, carbohydrate, and fat calories to achieve your goals. Get ready; you're about to change your life!

Building Muscle and Burning Fat

Bodybuilding is a delicate balance between building muscle and burning fat. You need adequate calories to increase muscle mass, but you also need a caloric deficit to burn off stored fat. It sounds impossible, but it isn't. The secret? Basic math. Or, as it's referred to in the fitness world: the Energy Balance Equation. Simply put, the more muscle mass you have, and the more active you are, the more you need to eat. That's because the more lean muscle mass you have, the more energy (thanks, food!) it takes to move that muscle around. Anything from basic functions like breathing, digestion, and your heart beating, to walking around and carrying the laundry up the stairs, or more deliberate exercise like running or pushing serious weight in the gym—your body needs energy, and if you're doing all these tasks with more lean muscle, you need more fuel.

Before you go running to the fridge, let's look at the other end of the spectrum. When we eat more calories than our body uses, all those extra calories are stored as fat. This is the reason why many people who gorge to get strong, never actually become lean and shredded. They may indeed get stronger, but getting lean means cutting out extra calories. There are still other factors to consider, like poor food quality, lack of nutrient timing, and improper ratios of macronutrients. All calories are, of course, not created equal. We want to fuel our body with the best building blocks, at the right time to power our workout, improve our performance, grow more muscle, and get rid of extra body fat.

Let's start by looking at some of the best foods to help us achieve our goals.

THE FIFTEEN BEST MUSCLE-BUILDING FOODS

Ordered by protein content (greater to lesser), veggies, fruits, starches

1 **Beef from grass-fed cattle**, when compared to grain-fed beef, has a lower fat content, contains more essential fatty acids and antioxidants, and less of those fats that increase cholesterol.

2 **White meat**: chicken, turkey and pork are all great sources of lean white meat. Low in fat and high in protein, it allows you to get all the grams of protein you need without sending your caloric intake through the roof.

3 **Salmon** is one of the greatest food sources of vitamin D. Studies have proven that vitamin D contributes to greater muscular strength.

4 **Crustaceans** are wonderful sources of lean protein and zinc. Zinc is essential for physical exercise, and the more we exert, the more of it is depleted. Maintaining high levels of zinc will help you perform your best.

5 **Egg yolks** are high in cholesterol, the type of fat your body uses most effectively for building testosterone. They also provide vitamin D, a vitamin linked to higher testosterone levels. The trick, of course, is moderation, so watch your portions.

6 **Greek yogurt** has fewer carbohydrates and way more protein (23g a cup!) than regular yogurt, and provides probiotics that aide digestion and improve nutrient absorption.

7 **Beans** are the most budget-friendly protein you can buy. Besides protein, beans offer tons of fiber and slow-digesting carbohydrates that help stabilize blood sugar throughout your workout and everyday activities.

8 **Quinoa** is the only grain considered a complete protein. It provides essential amino acids, as well as vitamins, minerals, antioxidants, and fiber. Make sure to take its carb content into consideration when planning meals, however.

9 **Cruciferous vegetables** include broccoli, bok choy, cauliflower, cabbage, Brussels sprouts, radishes, kale, and collard greens, to name a few. These vegetables provide a natural source of aromatase inhibitors that help control estrogen and improve levels of free testosterone.

10 **Apples** contain ursolic acid, a natural compound that blocks certain types of mRNA related to muscle loss, and causes greater muscle growth by enhancing insulin-like growth factor 1 (IGF-1) signaling.

11 **Bananas** are a cheap and tasty carb source, full of potassium and fiber, that studies have proven to be just as effective in improving performance as carbohydrate drinks.

12 **Beets** are an excellent source of nitric oxide, a supplement proven to improve performance, fight fatigue, and provide a faster recovery. They are perfect as a pre-workout snack to bring out your best.

13 **Coconuts** contain a healthy source of testosterone-building saturated fats. Diets too low in saturated fat have been shown to cause a decrease in testosterone, which can limit your potential gains in the gym.

14 **Russet potatoes** are a fast-absorbing carb with a very high glycemic index. After an intense training session they will help refuel your muscle for the next workout, improving recovery and increasing your training load.

15 **Sweet potatoes** are the best source of beta-carotene, a powerful antioxidant that will help you put on muscle mass. It is proven to improve levels of insulin-like growth factor 1 (IFG-1), which promotes muscle growth and reduces protein breakdown.

THE FIFTEEN BEST FAT-BURNING FOODS

1 **Lean protein** is needed in higher than typical amounts when cutting calories to prevent the loss of lean mass. Sources of protein lower in overall calories, like shrimp, pork loin, chicken breasts, egg whites, or nonfat Greek yogurt, would be the best choice for weight loss.

2 **Cold water fish** have large amounts of omega-3 fatty acids that have been shown to improve levels of leptin, a hormone that helps regulate your sense of hunger and fullness.

3 **Nuts** are high in protein, fiber, and healthy fats. Clinical trials have shown that low-calorie diets that include nuts lead to greater weight loss than diets lacking nuts. They are also calorie-dense, however, so be mindful of your portion sizes!

4 **Cruciferous vegetables** provide disease-fighting phytochemicals. One in particular, indole-3-carbinol, helps weight loss, fights weight gain, improves glucose tolerance, and helps regulate levels of estrogen and testosterone.

5 **Spinach,** and other green-plant membranes like it, are proven to be an important part of diets, causing significant weight loss, improving cholesterol levels, decreasing the urge to eat sweets, and helping curb hunger.

6 **Hot peppers** are packed with a compound called *capsaicin* that helps reduce appetite. Also, by stimulating the body's sympathoadrenal system, they intensify metabolism so you can burn more calories from stored fat.

7 **Apples.** In a recent study, apple pectin was shown to prevent weight gain and fat storage by strengthening gut barrier function, improving the balance of bacteria in the digestive tract, and relieving inflammation. Like other sources of soluble fiber, apple pectin also improves cholesterol levels and heart health.

8 **Citrus fruit** is full of vitamin C, antioxidants, flavonoids, and the soluble fiber pectin. Grapefruit, specifically, contains naringenin, an antioxidant that improves the body's use of insulin and increases calorie burn. Studies have also found that after ingesting p-synephrine, found in bitter orange, the body will use more of its fat stores to fuel exercise.

9 **Raspberries.** Raspberry ketone is a natural phenolic compound found in red raspberry. Not only does raspberry ketone help prevent weight gain, it also increases the breakdown of stored fat in the body.

10 **Whole rolled oats and oat bran** are rich in the water-soluble fiber beta-glucan, which improves cholesterol levels and improves heart health. Oats are also slow-digesting, so you feel full and satisfied longer than with other cereals.

11 **Cinnamon** helps regulate blood sugar. Adding cinnamon to your diet can reduce insulin resistance brought on by poor dietary habits, and can counteract the negative effects stress has on weight gain.

12 **Psyllium husk** is a low-calorie source of fiber. When it comes in contact with water, it swells, so adding it to any meal makes the meal itself denser and filling, so you can maintain your caloric goals.

13 **Apple cider vinegar** has been proven to improve cholesterol levels when taken regularly. Vinegar in general, when part of a meal, can reduce spikes in blood sugar so you feel full and satisfied longer.

14 **Green tea** contains catechins and caffeine that increase energy metabolism, leading to weight loss. When they work together, the thermogenesis of fat is even and exercise-induced loss of abdominal fat is greater.

15 **Coconut oil** is digested differently than other fats. Its breakdown helps improve energy metabolism and protects the liver from damage. Daily supplementation of coconut oil specifically helps reduce abdominal fat and improves cholesterol levels.

THE NINE PRINCIPLES OF THE BODYBUILDING DIET

Eating well isn't rocket science. Incorporating these nine simple principles is a fast way to fix your eating habits and get started on the right path to reaching your goals.

1. Plan Well

Eating for gains takes planning. Before leaving your house, have a grocery list laying out what and how much you need to buy to prepare all your food for the next week. Plan out your portions. Prep your meals. Have them ready in food containers, ready to travel with you in a lunch box, with ice packs that can keep it cold all day. Even if your goal is just to be healthy, regardless of whether or not you have a rippling six-pack, planning ahead is the only way to make it happen.

It may seem like prepping your food takes a lot a time, but in reality it saves you time. It is less stressful, it's often cheaper than getting takeout, and it works. Take the time to plan well and, I promise, your results will astound you.

2. Count Your Calories

Counting calories is by far the fastest and most effective way to identify and eliminate problems with your diet. Record just a few days of your diet and you will see exactly what is limiting your results. Most people quickly realize that they aren't eating nearly enough protein, and every so often someone discovers that they are consuming so little that it is actually hampering their results.

If you monitor both your activity level and the calories you need to fuel that activity, you'll end up feeling great. Going on vacation or off your routine, or going out to a restaurant or being social with your friends will no longer be a problem. If you have never counted calories before, try for a short period of time to get a baseline of where you are, and an idea of what you need to adjust to achieve your goals.

3. Protein, Protein, Protein!

Protein is crucial to adding new muscle and preserving the muscle you have, but the benefits don't stop there. Higher protein diets are associated with increased thermogenesis—turning your body into a fat burning machine. Moderately high-protein diets can stimulate muscle protein anabolism, or building of new muscle fibers, so more muscle mass is maintained and your metabolic rate is greater. Protein by itself will improve your sense of satiety, so you are left feeling full and satisfied longer, making it easier to stick to your diet. These incredible benefits mean greater fat loss and greater retention of muscle, so you end up jacked and shredded.

Now that we all agree we need protein, the real trick is getting enough. Studies in sports science recommend that athletes consume a minimum of 1.3 to 1.8 grams of protein per each kilogram of bodyweight. Elevated protein consumption—1.8 to 2 grams of protein per kilogram of body weight—may help prevent muscle loss when restricting calories to cut body fat. And for those doing resistance training while restricting calories, 2.3 to 3.1 grams of protein per kilogram of lean body weight is best. The greater the caloric restriction and leanness, the more protein is recommended.

If you're doing the math, you are probably thinking, "Wow...that's a lot of protein," and you are right. If you're not used to eating so much protein it might seem impossible to ingest hundreds of grams of protein each day, but you can, and it's easy, as long as you plan ahead. By incorporating protein into each meal, the totals add up quickly. Later we will discuss how to figure out your own protein needs so you can plan out your daily intake.

4. Eat Good Carbs

Carbs have been given a bad reputation that they don't truly deserve. Our body needs carbohydrates to function properly; we just want to make sure we choose the right ones. Carbohydrates found in fruit, vegetables, beans, nonfat dairy products, and whole grains come with valuable nutrients and fiber. Limiting these foods can impair electrolyte levels and cause, in the long run, deficiencies in essential vitamins, minerals, and fiber. These deficiencies can then have negative effects on your health and severely impair your results in the gym. When carbohydrates are restricted, fatigue occurs when muscle glycogen is depleted during bouts of exercise. Timing the right carbohydrates pre- and post-workout is definitely the best game plan for optimal performance and maximum results.

5. Stick to Healthy Fats

Healthy fats are an essential part of a healthy diet. Linoleic acid (LA), an omega-6 fatty acid, and α-linoleic acid (ALA), an omega-3 fatty acid, cannot be synthesized inside our body and therefore are considered essential fatty acids. If we don't consume enough through our diet, we become deficient. Foods that are rich in LA include plant sources like sunflower seeds, pecans, and sesame oil. Flaxseeds, chia seeds, and walnuts are among the richest dietary sources of ALA.

Fatty acids serve many purposes. Both omega-3 and omega-6 fatty acids are essential structural components of the cell membrane, are precursors to bioactive lipid mediators and hormones, and provide energy. Healthy levels are important for proper neurological and visual development and have shown a correlation to mood and mental function, especially as we age. And in terms of getting lean, diets high in protein and these specific types of fats have been shown to significantly improve overall body fat percentage.

6. Eat Your Veggies

Low in calories, high in fiber, and packed with the vitamins and minerals your body needs, vegetables are a nutritional cornerstone of any healthy diet. Compounds in vegetables provide an abundance of benefits to your overall body fat, gut health, immune functions, cardiovascular strength, complexion, energy levels, and mental well-being.

Vegetables provide nutrients that are critical to overall fitness and performance. Specific vegetables like beets and tomatoes boost endurance and speed up recovery by reducing exercise-induced stress on the body. Additionally, vegetables such as spinach and sweet potatoes are important sources of electrolytes. Vegetables are also key to keeping body fat low. Their filling fiber and low calories are a huge help when hunger strikes. Cell membranes in green plants and compounds in cruciferous vegetables help improve weight loss, prevent weight gain, and target problem areas by helping to regulate hormone levels. Eating a variety of vegetables throughout the day is an easy way to ensure you are getting a good mixture of all they can offer.

7. Avoid Processed Foods

Calorie for calorie, lower-quality foods like processed snacks, refined grains and sugars, fried foods, and food high in saturated and trans fats will accelerate weight gain. High-quality foods that are unrefined and minimally processed lead to a better overall body fat composition and a more shredded physique. High-quality foods include fresh vegetables and fruits, whole grains, healthy fats, and healthy sources of protein.

Buying whole foods and preparing them at home is the best way to ensure the quality of the foods you eat. Food labels should only list few ingredients that are easy to pronounce and recognize. For example, a canister of oats should have one ingredient: whole rolled oats. If you top it with fresh blueberries, a dash of sweetener, and a little unsweetened almond milk you have a delicious whole foods breakfast—much better than a packet of instant blueberry oatmeal, with a dozen ingredients, half of which are chemicals and food dyes we can't even pronounce.

8. Drink Water . . . Lots of It

Water is essential for life. Second to breathing, it is the one thing you can't go without. The majority of our body is water, and having enough of it is necessary for all cells, including our muscles, to function properly. When well-hydrated, the heart doesn't have to work as hard to pump blood to the body, and nutrients and oxygen are transported more efficiently to and from the muscles, so you have more energy and better endurance. A well-hydrated athlete will feel stronger and more powerful and have the ability to work out longer, harder, and more effectively.

During physical activity it's not uncommon for a person to sweat out 6 to 10 percent of their body weight. You want to replenish that loss, which can affect both physical and mental performance if ignored. Even mild dehydration reduces endurance, increases fatigue, reduces motivation, alters body temperature regulation, and makes exercises seem harder than usual. Rehydration can reduce these symptoms and lower the oxidative stress exercising puts on your body. Water needs vary based on size, activity, and temperature, so the rule of thumb is that *if you are thirsty, you have waited too long.* Carry water with you and sip it throughout the day. It is the first step to a killer workout.

9. Be Disciplined (Most of the Time)

Life is about balance, and there is a happy equilibrium where all of us can enjoy life and still get results. Being fit doesn't mean eating cardboard and forgoing all of life's pleasures so that you can be in the gym spinning on a hamster wheel. Discover ways to be active that get you excited. Make healthy choices most of the time, and stay mindful of moderation.

At times when socializing revolves around heavy eating and drinking alcoholic beverages, the onus is on you to focus on having fun that doesn't undermine your fitness goals. Be active with your friends, have healthy dinner parties at home instead of going to restaurants, and avoid celebrating with sweets. If you're only weeks away from a wedding or stepping on stage in a posing suit, you have no room for mistakes. But, during the rest of the time, assuming you stay in control, enjoying a goodie or two once in a while is okay. If you are not getting the results you're working for, that's a good indication that a little more discipline is needed.

WHAT YOU SHOULD EAT
PRE- AND POST-WORKOUT

Your performance and your results depend on what you eat before and in a window of time right after working out, so timing and ratios of macronutrients is really important. Getting it right allows for better recovery, increased muscle growth, and improved mood.

Recipes in the book have been labeled as either ideal for pre- or post-workout, giving you a leg up.

IDEAL FOR PRE-WORKOUT

Macronutrients ideal for pre-workout are protein, fat, and carbohydrates (slow-, fast-digesting, or both). In the meal you have just prior to working out, carbohydrates can improve endurance. Fast-digesting carbs can lead to rapid glycogen resynthesis, so if you are working out in the morning after a whole night of fasting, this might be the best way to get your muscles ready for the gym. Slow-digesting carbs have been shown to help increase fast oxidation during exercise, so if you are really trying to shed those last few pounds this is a better choice for you. Pre-workout meals higher in fat may enhance fat oxidation, and consuming protein before resistance training can maximize the synthesis of new muscle. Finally, caffeine and dietary nitrates, like those in beet juice, seem to enhance performance.

IDEAL FOR POST-WORKOUT

Macronutrients ideal for post-workout are protein and fast-digesting carbohydrates. Eating protein, alongside resistance training, is a powerful stimulus for muscle growth, and a key factor in regulating muscle mass. Within 30 minutes of finishing your workout, consuming a high dose of carbohydrates has been shown to stimulate glycogen resynthesis, and may stimulate even greater volumes of protein synthesis in your muscles.

How to Make It All Work for Your Goals

The key to finding a successful meal plan is to figure out what *your* body needs, and give it exactly that. Follow the steps below to determine the caloric and protein needs for your unique goals.

1. CALCULATE YOUR FAT-FREE MASS USING SKINFOLD THICKNESS

Taking the time to figure out your fat-free mass takes a bit more effort than just stepping on a scale, but it is absolutely essential for getting the results you want. Your fat free mass (FFM), or lean mass, is the amount of body weight that is not fat (muscle, bone, organs, etc.) and is thus productive, therefore needing calories to perform throughout the day. Body fat predictors like Body Mass Index (BMI), which simply compare height and weight, are inaccurate for muscular individuals. For this reason, any calculation that predicts your caloric needs based on gender, age, height, and weight alone are not effective. Scales or handheld devices that calculate FFM using bioelectrical impedance are also incredibly inaccurate.

The most effective (and, it turns out, cost-effective) way to calculate your FFM is skinfold thickness. I recommend using a method that takes at least seven skinfold measurements into account (a quick online search will pull up all the sites). Purchase calipers and then have a friend help you measure any hard to reach places. If you are not confident in your technique, ask a certified trainer at a gym to help you out. Once you have all the numbers, punch them into any one of the many online calculators to find your percentage of fat mass.

Once you know your overall body weight and percentage fat mass, you can easily find your FFM.

Body Weight x Percentage Fat Mass = Fat Mass

Body Weight – Fat Mass = **Fat Free Mass**

2. CALCULATE YOUR CALORIC NEEDS

Your caloric need is a combination of your BMR (Basal Metabolic Rate, also known as Resting Metabolic Rate) and your activity level. The Katch-McArdle equation factors in a person's FFM and is the preferred method for those with an above average amount of muscle.

BMR = 370 + (9.8 x FFM in pounds)

or

BMR = 370 + (21.6 x FFM in kilograms)

Calorie expenditure will vary based on your activity throughout the day. This includes both deliberate exercise and everyday tasks. Multiply your BMR by the appropriate Physical Activity Factor to estimate your daily caloric needs:

Little to no exercise   BMR x 1.2

Light exercise (1–3 days per week)   BMR x 1.375

Moderate exercise (3–5 days per week)   BMR x 1.55

Heavy exercise (6–7 days per week)   BMR x 1.725

Very heavy exercise (twice per day, extra heavy workouts)   BMR x 1.9

= Daily Caloric Need To Maintain Weight

Consuming the amount of calories that matches your daily caloric need will allow you to maintain your weight. If your goal is to lose body fat, you want to set your calorie allowance slightly lower. To maintain muscle, this calorie restriction should not be set to lose more than one percent of your body weight per week. A calorie deficit of 500 calories a day would result in about 1 pound of weight loss a week. Conversely, if your goal is to add muscle mass, you need to set your calorie allowance just slightly higher to provide extra fuel for muscles to build. Generally 125 to 250 extra calories a day is adequate. If your current daily intake is far from this amount, make gradual changes every few days to move your caloric intake in the right direction. But beware: increasing or decreasing your calories all at once can have adverse effects on weight gain or energy levels. Keep an eye on your progress: as your body changes and you put on more muscle mass, these calculations will need to be readjusted.

Daily Caloric Allowance =

Daily Caloric Needs to Maintain +/- adjustment to lose or gain

3. CALCULATE YOUR MACRONUTRIENT NEEDS

Within your daily caloric allowance lies an important balance of macronutrients. Studies show that to maintain muscle in a resistance training program while restricting calories, you need to consume 2.3 to 3.1 grams of protein per kilogram of fat-free mass. Fifteen to thirty percent of total calories should come from healthy fat, and the remainder from good carbohydrates. Use the following equations to calculate how many grams of each macronutrient you need each day. The examples here calculate using high-end requirements. If you prefer to find your low end, swap out the numbers accordingly.

Protein:

FFM in kilograms x 3.1 g = **grams of protein needed each day**

or

FFM in pounds x 1.41 g = **grams of protein needed each day**

Fat:

Daily calorie allowance x 0.3 = daily calories from fat

Daily calories from fat / 9 = **grams of fat needed each day**

Carbohydrates:

Daily calorie allowance – daily calories from fat –
(4 x grams of protein needed each day) = daily calories from carbohydrates

Daily calories from carbohydrates / 4 = **grams of carbohydrates needed each day**

4. PICK THE RECIPES THAT FIT YOUR BODY'S NEEDS

Now that you know how many grams of protein, fat, and carbohydrate to eat each day, the rest is easy! Look at the nutritional value of the recipes in the book, all conveniently listed upfront in the table of contents, and pick in the ones that fit your daily needs and mood. If you aren't sure where to start, chapter 2 will get you going with some meal plans. All the recipes throughout the book are labeled as either MB or FB. Here's why:

- **MB—Muscle Building:** Compared to the amount of protein, these recipes have a higher amount of fat and carbohydrates. If you are trying to shed pounds of fat, too many MB recipes make it challenging to get all your protein for the day without going over your daily calorie allowance. These recipes also tend to include items on the *15 Best Muscle Building Food* list, and are a good choice for pre- or post-workout.

- **FB—Fat Burning:** Compared to the amount of protein, these recipes have a lower amount of fat and carbohydrates. If you are trying shed pounds of fat, FB recipes make it easy to get all your protein for the day without going over your daily calorie allowance. These recipes also tend to include items on the *15 Best Fat Burning Foods* list.

CHAPTER TWO

PLANNING AHEAD

WEEKLY MEAL PLANS

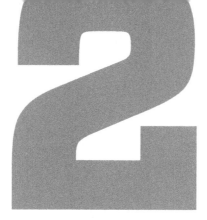

In chapter 1, we set the groundwork for building your meal plan, discussed how to calculate your daily caloric needs, and discussed how to determine the breakdown of macronutrients in grams of protein, carbohydrates, and fats. Whichever recipes you choose and whatever flavors you prefer, just make sure that the numbers add up. Make sure to have protein in each meal, adjust the portions in relation to your caloric allowance, and time your pre- and post-workout meals thoughtfully.

This chapter puts it all together with sample weekly meals. Each sample week indicates potential workout times each day (early morning, mid morning, midday, afternoon, evening, double days, and rest days) that will help you picture your own schedule (or work out a new one), also showing how recipes prepared in bulk can carry over across several days if bulk preparation is your thing. You may prefer to eat a different selection every day, and that's also fine. The point is to find something that fits your life, is on track with your goals, and satisfies your taste buds.

Muscle Building

If your goal is to put on muscle mass, set your caloric allowance a little *higher* than your daily caloric need for maintenance. Generally, 125 to 250 extra calories is adequate.

REST DAY

Crab Cakes 56

Oatmeal Cookie Bars 254

Shrimp Creole 149

Turkey Stroganoff 82

Pot Roast 118/
Savory Roasted Cauliflower 195

Greek Yogurt "Cheesecake" 216

DAY 1

Nuts About Honey Shake 245

EARLY MORNING WORKOUT

Almond Butter and Honey Crisps 257

Shrimp Creole 149

Pot Roast 118/
Savory Roasted Cauliflower 195

Honey-Dijon Kale Salad
(with chicken) 184

Greek Yogurt "Cheesecake" 216

DAY 2

Overnight Oats 44/
Eggs to Go 42

Blueberries and Beets Smoothie 244

MORNING WORKOUT

Almond Butter and Honey Crisps 257

Pot Roast 118/
Savory Roasted Cauliflower 195

Broiled Salmon with Indian Spices 172/
Curry Quinoa Salad 189

Greek Yogurt "Cheesecake" 216

DAY 3

Overnight Oats 44/
Eggs to Go 42

Cabbage Rolls 106

Blueberries and Beets Smoothie 244

MIDDAY WORKOUT

Almond Butter and Honey Crisps 257

Eye Round Steak 113/
Thai Peanut Salad 188

Greek Yogurt "Cheesecake" 216

MB

DAY 4

Overnight Oats 44/
Eggs to Go 42

Cabbage Rolls 106

Slow Cooker Beef Stew 119

Eye Round Steak 113/
Quinoa with Mushrooms
and Spinach 202

AFTERNOON WORKOUT

Almond Butter and Honey Crisps 257

Almond-Crusted Pork Cutlets 138/
Chunky Applesauce 205

DAY 5

Overnight Oats 44/
Eggs to Go 42

Cabbage Rolls 106

Slow Cooker Beef Stew 119

Orange Creamsicle Shake 248

Eye Round Steak 113/
Quinoa with Mushrooms
and Spinach 202

EVENING WORKOUT

Almond Butter and Honey Crisps 257

DAY 6

Nuts About Honey Shake 245

WORKOUT 1

Sloppy Joes
(served in a baked potato) 116

Eye Round Steak 113/
Quinoa with Mushrooms
and Spinach 202

WORKOUT 2

Almond Butter and Honey Crisps 257

Scallop Stir-Fry 158

Fat Burning

If your goal is to shed body fat, set your caloric allowance a little *lower* than your daily caloric need for maintenance. To maintain muscle while dropping fat, caloric restriction should be no more than one percent of your body weight per week. In general, a deficit of 500 calories a day should result in one pound of weight loss a week.

REST DAY

Banana Pancakes 48

Snickerdoodle Bars 252

Mahimahi Tacos 174

Pork Chile Verde 141

Turkey Satay Skewers 73/
Cucumber Salad 178

Key Lime Protein Pie 226

DAY 1

Raspberry-Orange Shake 249

EARLY MORNING WORKOUT

Apple Pie Pockets 222/
Protein Pumpkin-Spice Latte 237

Turkey Satay Skewers 73/
Cucumber Salad 178

Pork Chile Verde 141

Coconut Seared Scallops
with Wilted Spinach 156

Key Lime Protein Pie 226

DAY 2

Breakfast Casserole 53

Banana Bread Bars 266

MORNING WORKOUT

Apple Pie Pockets 222/
Protein Pumpkin-Spice Latte 237

Turkey Satay Skewers 73/
Cucumber Salad 178

Crispy Chicken with
Sweet Mustard Dip 70

Key Lime Protein Pie 226

DAY 3

Breakfast Casserole 53

Go Nuts Granola
(on Greek yogurt) 45

Banana Bread Bars 266

MIDDAY WORKOUT

Apple Pie Pockets 222/
Protein Pumpkin-Spice Latte 237

Garlic and Rosemary Grilled
T-Bones 112/
Spinach Caprese Salad 185

Peaches 'n' Cream Shake 240

FB

DAY 4

Breakfast Casserole 53

Go Nuts Granola
(on Greek yogurt) 45

Snickerdoodle Bars 252

Citrus Beet Salad with
Toasted Walnuts 182/
Oven-Roasted Turkey Breast 87

AFTERNOON WORKOUT

Apple Pie Pockets 222/
Protein Pumpkin-Spice Latte 237

Peanut Chicken (with veggies) 90

DAY 5

Breakfast Casserole 53

Go Nuts Granola
(on Greek yogurt) 45

Snickerdoodle Bars 252

Citrus Beet Salad with
Toasted Walnuts 182/
Oven-Roasted Turkey Breast 87

Banana Bread Bars 266

EVENING WORKOUT

Chewy Gooey Fudge Bars 258/
Root Beer Float Shake 246

DAY 6

Raspberry-Orange Shake 249

WORKOUT 1

Apple Pie Pockets 222/
Protein Pumpkin-Spice Latte 237

Citrus Beet Salad with
Toasted Walnuts 182/
Oven-Roasted Turkey Breast 87

WORKOUT 2

Chewy Gooey Fudge Bars 258/
Root Beer Float Shake 246

Grilled Ono with Mango-
Pineapple Salsa 170

Maintaining Weight

If you're at your ideal weight and your goal is to maintain it, set your calories allowance to match the daily caloric needs.

REST DAY

Huevos Rancheros
Hash Brown Skillet 64

Strawberry Cheesecake Bars 269

Chicken and Veggie
One-Dish Wonder 92

Grilled Balsamic and Rosemary
Salmon (with Veggies) 173

Roasted Garlic–Stuffed Italian Baked
Chicken (with Veggies) 104

Sugar- and Gluten-Free
Peanut Butter Cookies 220

DAY 1

Blueberry Muffin Shake 247

EARLY MORNING WORKOUT

Chewy Sweet Cinnamon Bars 262/
Cinnamon and Sugar Shake 234

Chicken and Veggie
One-Dish Wonder 92

Mexian Carnitas
(as tacos with veggies) 132

Turkey Lettuce Wraps 96

Sugar- and Gluten-Free
Peanut Butter Cookies 220

DAY 2

Sweet Potato Bran Muffins 52/
Turkey Breakfast Sausage 58

Protein Pumpkin-Spice Latte 237

MORNING WORKOUT

Chewy Sweet Cinnamon Bars 262/
Cinnamon and Sugar Shake 234

Chicken and Veggie
One-Dish Wonder 92

Apple and Oats Meatloaf
(with veggies) 117

Lemon Bar Cookie 267

DAY 3

Sweet Potato Bran Muffins 52/
Turkey Breakfast Sausage 58

Lemon Bar Cookie 267

Mexican Carnitas
(over rice with avocado) 132

MIDDAY WORKOUT

Chewy Sweet Cinnamon Bars 262/
Cinnamon and Sugar Shake 234

Ham and Bean Soup 139

Root Beer Float Shake 246

DAY 4

Sweet Potato Bran Muffins 52/
Turkey Breakfast Sausage 58

Lemon Bar Cookie 267

Apple and Oats Meatloaf
(with veggies) 117

Kung Pow Chicken 84/
Forbidden Fried Rice 198/
Stir-Fried Broccoli with Garlic 206

AFTERNOON WORKOUT

Hawaiian-Style Pork and
Pineapple Skewers 142

Peanut Butter–Nutella Shake 243

DAY 5

Sweet Potato Bran Muffins 52/
Turkey Breakfast Sausage 58

Lemon Bar Cookie 267

Apple and Oats Meatloaf
(with veggies) 117

Kung Pow Chicken 84/
Stir-Fried Broccoli with Garlic 206

Mexican Carnitas
(over rice with avocado) 132

EVENING WORKOUT

Hawaiian-Style Pork and
Pineapple Skewers 142

DAY 6

Blueberry Muffin Shake 247

WORKOUT 1

Apple and Oats Meatloaf
(with veggies) 117

Kung Pow Chicken 84/
Forbidden Fried Rice 198/
Stir-Fried Broccoli with Garlic 206

WORKOUT 2

Hawaiian-Style Pork and
Pineapple Skewers 142

Sugar- and Gluten-Free
Peanut Butter Cookies 220

Quick & Easy

This is a selection of recipes that can be whipped up in minutes, or prepared in bulk, and enjoyed for several days.

REST DAY

Steak and Eggs Omelet 60

Wild Berry Smoothie 236

Spicy Turkey Stir-Fry 78

Tuna Salad 161

Southwestern Salad
with Pulled Chicken 187

Chocolate Protein Mug Cake 230

DAY 1

Banana-Nut Muffin Shake 235

EARLY MORNING WORKOUT

Chocolate–Peanut Butter
Crispy Bars 260

Spicy Turkey Stir-Fry 78

Tuna Salad 161

Chicken Tortilla Soup 86

Chocolate Protein Mug Cake 230

DAY 2

Eggs to Go 42

Oats to Go 43

Peaches 'n' Cream Shake 240

MORNING WORKOUT

Chocolate–Peanut Butter
Crispy Bars 260

Spicy Turkey Stir-Fry 78

Southwestern Salad
with Pulled Chicken 187

Coconut Macaroons 224

DAY 3

Eggs to Go 42

Oats to Go 43

Peanut Butter Cup Bars 268

Your Mom's Herb Chicken 80/
Brussels Sprouts and Berries Salad 180

MIDDAY WORKOUT

Chocolate–Peanut Butter
Crispy Bars 260

Orange Beef 128

Coconut Macaroons 224

MF/TS

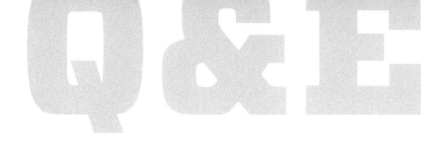

DAY 4

Eggs to Go 42

Oats to Go 43

Peanut Butter Cup Bars 268

Pulled Chicken
(as taco with veggies) 72

Orange Creamsicle Shake 248

AFTERNOON WORKOUT

Your Mom's Herb Chicken 80/
Protein Mashed Potatoes 196/
Garlicky Roasted Brussels Sprouts 192

Coconut Macaroons 224

DAY 5

Eggs to Go 42

Oats to Go 43

Peanut Butter Cup Bars 268

Pulled Chicken
(as taco with veggies) 72

Your Mom's Herb Chicken 80/
Brussels Sprouts and Berries Salad 180

15-Minute Beef Chili 115

EVENING WORKOUT

Protein Pineapple Jell-O Dessert 228

DAY 6

Banana-Nut Muffin Shake 235

WORKOUT 1

Protein Pineapple Jell-O Dessert 228

Honey-Garlic Shrimp
(with quinoa and veggies) 152

WORKOUT 2

Your Mom's Herb Chicken 80/
Protein Mashed Potatoes 196/
Garlicky Roasted Brussels Sprouts 192

Coconut Macaroons 224

MF/TS

CHAPTER THREE

BREAKFAST

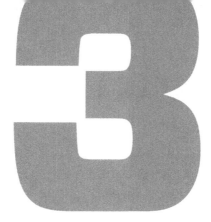

You've heard it before, and I'll say it again: Breakfast is the most important meal of the day. Your body is running on fumes after a full night's sleep, and breakfast is the first step to refueling, mentally and physically. Not only that, but skipping breakfast can seriously impair your gains. By missing this first important meal, every meal you eat during the rest of the day is metabolized less effectively, and the various hormones that control the sense of fullness and appetite are completely thrown off balance. So, although it may seem logical that missing a meal would be great for fat loss, this couldn't be less true. Skipping breakfast can actually lead to a greater Body Mass Index (BMI) and risk of developing Type II Diabetes. It can also increase the levels of the stress hormone cortisol, leading to weight gain and higher blood pressure.

The nutritional makeup of that daily meal is very important. Breakfasts high in protein make weight management much easier. Protein first thing in the morning helps control hunger throughout the day; it reduces cravings, making it easier to stick to your meal plan; and it improves your metabolism. Whether you are running out the door or sitting down for Sunday brunch, this chapter lists the best high-protein breakfasts that will get your day started just right.

MB Muscle Building **FB** Fat Burning **D-F** Dairy-Free **LC** Low Carb **G-F** Gluten-Free **P** Paleo **V** Vegan

EGGS TO GO

SERVES 1 / PREP TIME: 3 MINUTES / COOK TIME: 3 MINUTES

Ideal for batch cooking

This is an excellent go-to breakfast for those rushed mornings on the way to work. Nicely complemented with a serving of Oats to Go (page 43), the fluffy protein-packed egg whites and wake-you-up zing of salsa are the perfect way to start the day. Glamorous it may not be, but who cares when it is quick, portable and, most importantly, delicious.

Extra-virgin olive oil spray

5 egg whites

2 teaspoons diced bell pepper

2 teaspoons diced red onion

2 tablespoons salsa or a
   drizzle sriracha

Ingredient tip: *If you like your eggs plain, leave out the veggies.*

Time-saving tip: *Prepare a few days' worth of the egg, pepper, and onion at a time. Refrigerate portions separately in airtight microwave-safe storage containers, remove as needed, and microwave. Then add the garnish of your choice.*

1 Lightly spray a 2-cup microwave-safe storage container with olive oil spray. Add the egg whites, bell pepper, and onion to the container. Seal and refrigerate until you are ready to prepare.

2 To prepare the eggs, loosen the container lid so steam can vent. Microwave on high for 2 minutes. Shake the container gently. If the egg whites are still runny, microwave for 1 minute more in 15-second increments, checking for doneness after each increment, until cooked through. Cooking time may vary based on the depth and width of the storage container.

3 Garnish with salsa, and enjoy.

| FB | D-F | LC | G-F | P |

PER SERVING

Calories **145** Carbohydrates **2g** Fat **0g** Protein **25g**

OATS TO GO

SERVES 1 / PREP TIME: 2 MINUTES / COOK TIME: 1 MINUTE

Ideal for batch cooking • Ideal for pre-workout

This is a great companion to Eggs to Go (page 42). Together, they're an especially satisfying combination to start the morning with. This recipe opts for oat bran over oatmeal because the fiber content is a bit higher, the carbohydrates a little bit lower, and the texture a whole lot better—but you could definitely use whole rolled oats instead.

⅓ cup oat bran

1½ teaspoons granulated stevia

1½ teaspoons ground cinnamon

½ scoop whey protein powder, vanilla or cinnamon flavor

½ cup water

Ingredient tips: Go ahead and mix up the ratios of oats to protein to best suit your caloric needs. You could go 100 percent oats with no protein powder, or up the protein to a full scoop. Either way it will taste delicious. You will need to adjust the amount of water based on changes to the ingredients.

Nutritional information may vary based on the brand of protein you are using.

1 In a 1¼ cup microwave-safe storage container, combine the oat bran, stevia, cinnamon, and whey protein powder. Seal the lid, and store in the pantry until you are ready to prepare.

2 To cook, add the water and stir. Place the lid on loosely to allow steam to vent. Microwave on high for 1 minute.

3 Stir and enjoy.

Time-saving tip: Prepare a few days' worth of the dry ingredients at a time. Store portions separately in airtight microwave-safe storage containers, remove as needed, add water, and microwave. This is also a great recipe for making a double serving. Just double the ingredients and use a 2-cup container. You may need to microwave for 1 minute more.

MB **D-F** **G-F**

PER SERVING

Calories **141** Carbohydrates **22g** Fat **3g** Protein **18g**

OVERNIGHT OATS

SERVES 1 / PREP TIME: 5 MINUTES, PLUS 20 MINUTES TO CHILL

Ideal for pre-workout

Prepare this breakfast the night before so you can hit "snooze" in the morning. An easy no-bake recipe for complex carbs that's ready when you wake up. Enjoy it with some Eggs to Go (page 42), or an extra scoop of protein powder to punch up the protein content.

½ cup whole rolled oats

½ cup unsweetened vanilla almond milk or soy milk

2 tablespoons fresh blueberries or raspberries

1 tablespoon toasted and crushed walnuts or almonds (see page 182)

1 teaspoon granulated stevia

Dash ground cinnamon (optional)

1 In a 2-cup storage container or bowl, mix well to combine the oats, almond milk, berries, nuts, stevia, and cinnamon (if using). Cover and refrigerate for at least 20 minutes and up to overnight.

2 Enjoy cold.

Ingredient tip: You could also use frozen berries instead of fresh. Just soak them overnight first to defrost. If you want to up the protein, stir in a scoop of vanilla casein protein powder. Just remember to add your protein powder's calories to the total here.

MB **G-F** **V**

PER SERVING

Calories **231** Carbohydrates **31g** Fat **9g** Protein **8g**

GO NUTS GRANOLA

MAKES: 7 CUPS / PREP TIME: 10 MINS / COOK TIME: 25 MINS / TOTAL TIME: 50 MINS

Ideal for batch cooking

You will go nuts for this granola! Its nutritional profile is pretty amazing, giving you the essential fatty acids you need to start your day right. Paired with the fiber goodness of whole-rolled oats and a touch of cinnamon, this granola serves up a whole lot of yumminess. Enjoy with some soy milk or on top of some Greek yogurt, if you like.

¼ cup coconut oil, melted

¼ cup maple syrup or honey

1 teaspoon vanilla extract

3 cups whole rolled oats

1 cup shredded coconut

1 cup almonds, sliced, slivered, or chopped

1 cup cashews, chopped

1 cup walnuts, chopped

1 to 2 tablespoons ground cinnamon

2 tablespoons granulated stevia (optional)

Serving tip: This recipe makes a lot of granola, so be mindful of your portion sizes. Nuts are healthy, but they are also calorie-dense. A ¼ cup serving would make a good yogurt topper. A ½ cup topped with some almond or soy milk would make a good granola breakfast.

1 Preheat the oven to 325°F.

2 In a small bowl, mix together the coconut oil, maple syrup, and vanilla. Pour into 9-by-13-inch baking pan.

3 Add the oats, coconut, almonds, cashews, and walnuts, and mix again. Stir in the cinnamon and stevia (if using) until everything is evenly coated.

4 Press the granola mixture firmly down into the pan, and bake for 20 to 25 minutes, checking frequently after 15 minutes, until the granola is golden brown.

5 Remove from the oven, and cool for 15 minutes or more.

6 Break the granola up into chunks and serve.

MB　　　　　　　**G-F**　　**V**

PER SERVING

Calories **156**　Carbohydrates **11.8g**　Fat **11.4g**　Protein **3.9g**

¼ cup

SWEET POTATO LATKES
WITH CANDIED WALNUTS

MAKES 6 LATKES + 2 CUPS CANDIED WALNUTS / PREP TIME: 10 MINUTES / COOK TIME: 15 MINUTES

These sweet and savory sweet potato latkes, paired with candied walnuts, are a delicious way to start the morning. Especially with the good-for-you beta-carotene in sweet potatoes, and omega-3 essential fatty acid alpha-linolenic acid (ALA) in walnuts. What more could you need? If you want a bit more protein, these go perfectly with Turkey Breakfast Sausage (page 58).

FOR THE CANDIED WALNUTS

¼ cup granulated stevia

1 egg white

1 tablespoon water

2 cups raw walnuts, halved or chopped

1 teaspoon ground cinnamon

½ teaspoon salt

¼ teaspoon ground ginger

¼ teaspoon ground nutmeg

FOR THE SWEET POTATO LATKES

2 cups shredded raw sweet potato

3 egg whites

½ teaspoon ground cinnamon

¼ teaspoon ground nutmeg

⅛ teaspoon salt (optional)

Extra-virgin olive oil spray

TO MAKE THE CANDIED WALNUTS

1 Preheat the oven to 300°F.

2 In a medium bowl, whisk together the stevia, egg white, and water until frothy. Add the walnuts, and toss to coat.

3 Sprinkle the cinnamon, salt, ginger, and nutmeg over the walnuts, and toss to coat evenly.

4 Spread the walnuts on a foil-lined baking sheet in a single layer, and bake for 15 minutes.

MB **G-F** **P** **V**

PER SERVING

Calories **177** Carbohydrates **20g** Fat **9g** Protein **5g**

(2 latkes and 7 candied walnut halves)

TO MAKE THE SWEET POTATO LATKES

1 While the walnuts bake, in a medium bowl, use a fork to toss the sweet potatoes with the egg whites, cinnamon, nutmeg, and salt (if using) until well blended.

2 Heat a large skillet over medium heat, and lightly coat with olive oil spray. Scoop ⅓ cup of the latke mixture into the skillet, and flatten with a spatula. Repeat with the remaining mixture, working in batches if needed to avoid crowding the skillet. Cook for 4 minutes, flip, and cook for an additional 4 minutes.

3 Plate two latkes on each plate, top each serving with seven candied walnuts halves (0.5 ounce), and serve.

Time-saving tip: Candied walnuts can be prepared in bulk. These walnuts are great to have on hand, so double—or even triple—the ingredients and make as much as you want. You'll still have leftovers if you just make the candied walnuts as described here.

Ingredient tip: The latkes are best prepared fresh. This is a great recipe for scaling the ingredients up or down to increase or decrease the number of latkes made. The sweet potatoes can be peeled or not. Shred them in a food processor, or by hand using a grater.

Serving tip: You can top the latkes with some sugar-free maple syrup or real maple syrup. Just remember to add maple syrup's calories to the tally.

BANANA PANCAKES

MAKES 4 PANCAKES / PREP TIME: 5 MINUTES / COOK TIME: 10 MINUTES

This is the best protein pancake out there! The magic is in the psyllium husk that's in the pancake mix. The results are amazing, believe me. Not only does psyllium husk add a ton of fiber to clear out the pounds of protein we eat every day, it also really enhances the pancake-like texture. Fluffy and sweet, with just the slightest hint of banana and enough protein and fiber to keep you full all morning, you'll love them—guaranteed!

2 tablespoons psyllium husk
6 tablespoons water
1 ripe banana
2 whole eggs
¼ teaspoon vanilla extract
⅛ teaspoon baking soda
2 scoops whey protein, vanilla or cinnamon flavor
Extra-virgin olive oil spray

1 In a small bowl, mix the psyllium husk and water. Set aside.

2 Peel the banana, and put it in a medium bowl. Mash with a fork until mostly smooth. Add the psyllium husk slurry, eggs, vanilla, and baking soda, and stir until mostly smooth. Add the protein powder, and stir until a relatively smooth batter forms.

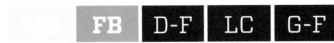

FB **D-F** **LC** **G-F**

PER SERVING

Calories **126** Carbohydrates **8.3g** Fat **3.3g** Protein **15.8g**

1 pancake

3 Heat a medium skillet over medium heat, and lightly coat with olive oil spray. Pour one-quarter of the batter into the pan, forming a cake about 8 inches in diameter. Let it cook undisturbed for about 1 minute, until many tiny bubbles form on top. Flip the pancake, and cook for about 1 minute more, until cooked through and the center is no longer runny.

4 Remove from the skillet, repeat with the remaining batter, and serve.

Ingredient tips: *Psyllium husk can be found in the bulk food section or health food aisle of most grocery stores.*

Not all protein powder is created equal, so choose your brand wisely. It will affect the taste, texture, and nutrition of the pancakes.

Lastly, for the bananas, you want the gross-looking brown ones you are about to throw away. Truly.

Serving tips: *Eat the pancakes plain or garnish as you like. For a low-calorie topping, try a sugar-free maple syrup. If you don't mind adding a few calories, melted peanut butter, banana slices, chopped walnuts, or honey are all delicious.*

PUMPKIN PIE PANCAKES

MAKES 4 PANCAKES / PREP TIME: 10 MINUTES / COOK TIME: 20 MINUTES

The almond flour and flax seed in these low-carb pancakes will keep you satisfied for hours, while giving your body the essential fatty acids it needs. Added bonus: the irresistible, fragrant scent of warm pumpkin pie that will fill your house.

½ cup almond flour

2 tablespoons milled flaxseed

2 tablespoons whey protein powder, vanilla or cinnamon flavor

1½ teaspoons ground cinnamon

¼ teaspoon ground allspice

¼ teaspoon ground cloves

¼ teaspoon ground ginger

¼ teaspoon ground nutmeg

¼ teaspoon baking soda

Pinch salt

¾ cup egg whites

½ cup canned pumpkin

2 tablespoons granulated stevia

½ teaspoon vanilla extract

1 teaspoon coconut oil

1 In a small bowl, mix together the almond flour, flaxseed, protein powder, cinnamon, allspice, cloves, ginger, nutmeg, baking soda, and salt.

2 In a medium bowl, mix together the egg whites, pumpkin, stevia, and vanilla until smooth.

3 Gradually stir the dry ingredients into the wet ingredients until smooth.

4 In a large skillet over medium heat, heat the coconut oil, swirling to coat the bottom.

5 Spoon one-quarter of the batter into the skillet, spreading the batter with the spoon to create the pancake, as it will be thick.

FB   D-F   LC   G-F   P

PER SERVING

Calories **122** Carbohydrates **5.5g** Fat **7g** Protein **10g**

1 pancake

6 Cook for about 3 minutes, until firm enough to flip. Cook an additional 2 minutes, and remove from the skillet. Repeat with the remaining batter.

7 Serve the pancakes plain or with the topping of your choice. Try a drizzle of honey and a sprinkle of roasted walnuts (note that these added toppings are not reflected in the nutritional breakdown here).

Ingredient tip: If you don't have almond flour on hand, you can make your own by grinding up whole almonds in a blender until they become flour.

SWEET POTATO BRAN MUFFINS

MAKES 4 MUFFINS / PREP TIME: 5 MINUTES / COOK TIME: 20 MINUTES

Ideal for pre-workout

A grab-and-go breakfast muffin made with beta-carotene-loaded sweet potatoes. All you need in one little muffin: carbs, protein, and healthy fats. Plenty of fiber and slow-digesting carbs to hold you over for several hours.

1½ cups (about 2½ medium) mashed, peeled, and baked sweet potato

2 eggs

1 teaspoon vanilla extract

½ cup oat bran

4 tablespoons casein protein powder, vanilla or cinnamon flavor (optional)

2 tablespoons granulated stevia

2 tablespoons psyllium husk

2 tablespoons milled flaxseed

1 teaspoon baking soda

1 teaspoon ground cinnamon

¼ teaspoon salt

4 teaspoons water (if using casein)

Ingredient tips: *Psyllium husk can be found in the bulk food section or health food aisle of most grocery stores.*

Sweet potatoes can be baked in the microwave in just a few minutes. Let them cool, scoop the meat out of the skin, and mash.

1 Preheat the oven to 325°F.

2 In a medium bowl, mix together the sweet potato, eggs, and vanilla.

3 In a separate medium bowl, mix together the oat bran, casein (if using), stevia, psyllium husk, milled flaxseed, baking soda, cinnamon, and salt.

4 Add the dry ingredients to the wet, adding the water if you added the casein, and stir. The batter will be thick.

5 Spoon the batter into a baking cup–lined muffin tin, dividing it evenly into 4 muffins.

6 Bake for 18 minutes, or until a toothpick inserted into the center comes out clean. Serve or store in the refrigerator for up to several days.

Time-saving tip: *This recipe scales up easily, so you can double or triple the ingredients for a larger batch of muffins.*

MB　　**D-F**　　**G-F**

PER SERVING

Calories **151** Carbohydrates **16.2g** Fat **6.5g** Protein **12.5g**

1 muffin w/ casein

BREAKFAST CASSEROLE

**SERVES 4 / PREP TIME: 20 MINUTES / COOK TIME: 1 HOUR /
TOTAL TIME: 1 HOUR, 30 MINUTES**

Just this one baking dish gets you a few days' worth of delicious breakfast. It travels and scales up pretty nicely, so you can take it along to a weekend brunch. Packed with protein, this oven-baked Western omelet is chock-full of juicy ham, tangy Greek yogurt, and bright red and green peppers for a tasty on-the-go breakfast.

Extra-virgin olive oil spray

6 egg whites, beaten

4 eggs, beaten

½ cup nonfat Greek yogurt

½ cup water

8 ounces fully cooked ham, cubed

½ cup (1 medium) diced green
   bell pepper

½ cup (1 medium) diced red
   bell pepper

½ cup (about 1 medium) diced onion

¼ cup (about 2) chopped green onion

1 Preheat the oven to 350°F.

2 Lightly coat an 8-inch-square baking dish with olive oil spray. Add the egg whites, eggs, yogurt, and water to the dish, and whisk until well-combined.

3 Stir in the ham, green and red bell peppers, onion, and green onion until all the ingredients are evenly spread throughout the casserole.

4 Bake for 45 to 60 minutes, until the eggs have set.

5 Remove from the oven and let rest for 10 minutes before cutting into 4 (4-by-4-inch) pieces and serving.

FB   LC   G-F

PER SERVING

Calories **197** Carbohydrates **6g** Fat **8.3g** Protein **24.8g**

1 square

FLOURLESS FAT-FREE CHEESE BLINTZES

MAKES 4 BLINTZES / PREP TIME: 10 MINUTES / COOK TIME: 15 MINUTES

A decadent brunch or dessert treat that has all the delicious flavor and creamy texture of a traditional blintz, without any flour or added sugar. Packed with protein, they can be prepped and ready to enjoy in a matter of minutes.

1 cup pasteurized egg whites (from a carton)

1 scoop casein protein powder, vanilla or cinnamon flavor

2 tablespoons granulated stevia, plus more as needed

1 cup fat-free cottage cheese

¼ cup fat-free ricotta cheese

1½ teaspoons freshly squeezed lemon juice

Extra-virgin olive oil spray

4 tablespoons sugar-free strawberry or raspberry jelly

1 In a blender or food processor, blend the egg whites, casein powder, and 2 tablespoons of stevia until smooth. (Alternatively, you can do this by hand in a medium bowl with a whisk.)

2 In a medium bowl, mix together the cottage cheese, ricotta, and lemon juice until the mixture is smooth.

3 Heat a large pan over medium-high heat, and lightly coat with olive oil spray.

FB **LC** **G-F**

PER SERVING

Calories **122** Carbohydrates **10.6g** Fat **0.4g** Protein **20.1g**

1 blintz

4 Pour ¼ cup of batter into the pan, and swirl the pan to create a thin layer. The circle should cover the surface area of the pan. The thinner the better. If you are new to making crepes, start with less than you would assume. You can add more to fill in holes, if needed.

5 As soon as the crepe is sturdy, flip it over and immediately spoon about ¼ cup of the cheese mixture onto the crepe in the lower quadrant nearest you. Fold the crepe over the filling. Then, fold in the two sides next to the filling, making an open-ended packet. Roll away from you as though making a little burrito. Let it sit only long enough to heat the filling, and remove from the pan. Repeat with the remaining batter.

6 In a small bowl, mix the jelly with a little bit of water so that it will have the consistency of a syrup or sauce. Add stevia if you prefer the dressing to be sweeter.

7 Spoon some of the fruit topping onto the blintzes, and serve immediately.

CRAB CAKES

**MAKES 4 CRAB CAKES / PREP TIME: 5 MINUTES /
COOK TIME: 10 MINUTES**

Ideal for pre-workout

Class up your breakfast act with some sweet, succulent crab cakes. A great balance of lean protein, healthy fats, and grain-free carbohydrates, this easy and quick dish will have you feeling like you're at a 5-star seafood restaurant.

2 tablespoons diced red onion

2 tablespoons diced celery

1 (6-ounce) can fancy crab meat or 4½ ounces fresh crab meat, thoroughly drained

2 tablespoons almond flour

2 tablespoons nutritional yeast

2 egg whites

¼ teaspoon mustard powder

Pinch ground paprika

Pinch ground cloves

Extra-virgin olive oil spray

1 In a small nonstick pan over medium heat, cook the onion and celery until soft, about 3 minutes. Transfer to a medium bowl.

2 Add the crab, almond flour, nutritional yeast, egg whites, mustard powder, paprika, and cloves to the bowl, and stir.

MB   D-F   G-F   P

PER SERVING

Calories **115** Carbohydrates **10.2g** Fat **4g** Protein **10g**

1 cake

3 Heat a large skillet over medium heat, and lightly coat with olive oil spray. Using your hands, form four cakes from the crab mixture. Place them in the skillet, and flatten with a spatula. Cook for about 3 minutes, until the bottom has browned and the cake is firm enough to flip. Flip the cakes and cook for 2 to 3 minutes more, until the bottom has browned and the cake is heated through.

4 Transfer to a plate and serve.

Ingredient tips: *Nutritional yeast is available online, in the bulk food section of many grocery stores, and in some health food aisles.*

If you don't have almond flour, you can make some by blending whole almonds into a flour.

Use egg whites from real eggs, as they hold together better than pasteurized egg whites from a carton.

Serving tips: *Some optional garnishes are chopped green onions, hot sauce, or a dollop of nonfat Greek yogurt. Just remember to add the extra calories to the recipe's nutritional breakdown.*

TURKEY BREAKFAST SAUSAGE

**MAKES 8 PATTIES / PREP TIME: 15 MINUTES, PLUS OVERNIGHT TO MARINATE /
COOK TIME: 5 MINUTES**

Ideal for batch cooking

Whipping up a batch of ultra-healthy lean protein sausages at home means
you have control over what goes in them: no extra crud like all the preservatives typically found in most store-bought varieties, just fresh ingredients.
Refrigerate these for three days, or freeze for up to three months.

1½ teaspoons salt

1½ teaspoons freshly ground
    black pepper

1 teaspoon fennel seed

1 teaspoon ground sage

1 teaspoon dried thyme

½ teaspoon garlic powder

Pinch ground cloves

Pinch onion powder

Pinch ground paprika

Pinch red pepper flakes

1½ teaspoons extra-virgin olive oil

1½ teaspoons maple syrup (optional)

1 pound 99% lean ground turkey

Extra-virgin olive oil spray

1 In a small bowl, mix together the salt,
black pepper, fennel, sage, thyme, garlic
powder, cloves, onion powder, paprika,
and red pepper flakes.

2 In a large bowl, drizzle the olive oil
and maple syrup (if using) over the
turkey, and mix well.

3 Sprinkle the spice mixture over the
turkey, and mix well.

FB **D-F** **LC** **G-F** **P**

PER SERVING

Calories **70** Carbohydrates **0.9g** Fat **1.4g** Protein **14g**

1 patty

4 Heat a small pan over medium-high heat, and lightly coat with olive oil spray. Using your hands, form one very small test patty. Cook until the bottom browns. Flip and continue cooking until brown and the center is no longer pink. Let the test patty cool enough to eat, and then sample it. At this point, if needed, adjust the spices to your liking in the raw ground turkey mix. Cover the bowl of turkey, and refrigerate overnight to allow the flavors to blend.

5 Using your hands, shape the turkey into 8 evenly sized patties.

6 Heat a large pan over medium-high heat, and lightly coat with olive oil spray. Cook for about 2 minutes, until the bottom browns. Flip and continue cooking until both sides are brown and the center is no longer pink, about 2 more minutes. Be careful not to overcook, or the sausages will be dry.

7 Serve immediately or freeze.

Time-saving tip: *Multiply this recipe to make as many servings as you want at once. Freeze them partially cooked, or cooked through, and reheat later.*

STEAK AND EGGS OMELET

SERVES 1 / PREP TIME: 5 MINUTES / COOK TIME: 10 MINUTES

Turn your dinner leftovers into a delicious omelet. Packed with muscle-building protein, colorful vegetables, and just enough egg yolk to benefit your hormone levels without giving your cardiologist a run for their money.

Extra-virgin olive oil spray

¼ cup (about ½ medium) diced onion

¼ cup (½ medium) diced bell pepper

2 cups chopped spinach

4 ounces High-Heat Eye of Round Roast (page 120), sliced into bite-size pieces

4 egg whites

1 egg

¼ cup (about ½ medium) diced tomato

Salt

Freshly ground black pepper

1 Heat an 8- to 10-inch nonstick skillet over medium heat, and very lightly coat with olive oil spray. Add the onion and bell pepper, and cook until the onion has softened, about 3 minutes.

2 Add the spinach and steak, and stir-fry until the spinach has wilted and the steak is heated through, about 2 minutes.

3 Transfer the steak and veggie mixture to a plate. If needed, wipe out the skillet. Return the skillet to medium heat.

4 In a blender or food processor, whip the egg white and egg for 45 seconds. You could also whip in a bowl by hand, but they will not be quite as fluffy.

MB   **D-F**   **G-F**   **P**

PER SERVING

Calories **373** Carbohydrates **12g** Fat **14g** Protein **48g**

5 Lightly coat the skillet in olive oil, pour the beaten eggs into the skillet, and swirl to coat the bottom of the pan. When the egg has partially set, about 1 to 2 minutes, use a spatula to scrape the edges and lift the egg so that the uncooked egg spreads to the hot cooking surface of the skillet.

6 Immediately lay the steak and veggie mixture and the tomato on one half of the omelet. Using a spatula, fold the empty half over the steak and veggies. Cook for about 2 minutes longer, until the eggs have set.

7 Plate the omelet, season with salt and pepper, and enjoy.

Ingredient tip: *Go ahead and use whatever meat you have on hand in the fridge. Nutrition will vary based on substitutions.*

Serving tip: *You may also enjoy garnishing the omelet with hot sauce, salsa, or a dollop of nonfat Greek yogurt.*

LEEK AND GOAT CHEESE FRITTATA

MAKES 6 SERVINGS / PREP TIME: 5 MINUTES / COOK TIME: 15 MINUTES

This savory frittata brings out perfectly the leeks' sweet flavor and tender texture. Goat cheese adds a deliciously tangy note, and has those filling fats that will keep you satisfied for hours.

1 tablespoon extra-virgin olive oil

3 large leeks, white and light green parts only, halved lengthwise and sliced ½ inch thick

Salt

4 large eggs

6 egg whites

Freshly ground black pepper

1 teaspoon chopped fresh thyme

2 ounces goat cheese, crumbled

Extra-virgin olive oil spray

1 Preheat the oven to 350°F.

2 In a 10-inch, ovenproof nonstick skillet over medium-high heat, heat the olive oil. Add the leeks, season with salt, and cook, stirring, until the leeks are tender and lightly browned, about 6 minutes. Transfer to a plate.

3 In a large bowl, whisk the eggs and egg whites. Season with pepper, add the leeks, thyme, and goat cheese, and gently stir to combine.

4 Wipe the skillet clean if needed, lightly coat with olive oil spray, and set over medium-low heat. Add the egg mixture to the pan, and gently shake the pan to evenly spread the mixture. Cook until the eggs begin to set around the edges, about 5 minutes, gently shaking the pan occasionally to be sure the frittata isn't sticking (if necessary, slide a spatula around the perimeter to release it).

5 Transfer the skillet to the oven, and bake until the center is set, about 5 minutes.

6 Remove from the oven and let rest for 2 minutes.

7 Carefully slide the frittata onto a serving plate, cut into six wedges, and serve warm.

MB **LC** **G-F**

PER SERVING

Calories **142** Carbohydrates **6.8g** Fat **7.3g** Protein **11.5g**

1 wedge

SMOKED SALMON SCRAMBLE

SERVES 1 / PREP TIME: 5 MINUTES / COOK TIME: 5 MINUTES

Why not start the day with vitamin D and protein-rich smoked salmon mingled into light and fluffy scrambled eggs?

1 tablespoon nonfat Greek yogurt

1 tablespoon water

4 egg whites

1 egg

¼ teaspoon fresh dill weed

Salt

Freshly ground black pepper

3 tablespoons chives, chopped, divided

Extra-virgin olive oil spray

2 ounces smoked salmon, cut into bite-size squares

Capers, for garnish (optional)

Fresh dill weed, for garnish (optional)

1 In a medium bowl, whisk the yogurt and water until smooth.

2 Add the egg whites and egg, and whisk until smooth.

3 Stir in the dill weed, season with salt and pepper, and stir in 2 tablespoons of chives.

4 Heat a medium skillet over medium-high heat, and lightly coat with olive oil spray. Pour the egg mixture into the skillet. Push cooked egg from the edges to the center of the skillet with a cooking spoon, and tip the skillet as necessary to get liquid egg in contact with the hot skillet. Continue until the eggs have come together but remain wet, about 3 minutes.

5 If you prefer your salmon warmed, stir in the salmon, cook for 1 minute more, and remove from the heat. If you prefer your salmon as a topping, cook the egg mixture for 1 minute more, transfer to a plate, and top with the smoked salmon.

6 Garnish with the remaining tablespoon of chives and the capers (if using) and dill (if using), and serve.

FB   **LC**   **G-F**

PER SERVING

Calories **246** Carbohydrates **2g** Fat **10g** Protein **35g**

HUEVOS RANCHEROS HASH BROWN SKILLET

SERVES 1 / PREP TIME: 5 MINUTES / COOK TIME: 15 MINUTES

Ideal for pre-workout • Ideal for post-workout

The fast-digesting russet potatoes quickly send energy to your muscles before or after your workout.

2 teaspoons extra-virgin olive oil, divided

½ cup shredded russet potato

⅛ teaspoon ground coriander, divided

2 dashes ground cayenne pepper, divided

2 dashes salt, divided

¼ cup black beans, rinsed and drained

2 tablespoons salsa

2 ounces Pulled Chicken (page 72) or Mexican Carnitas (page 132)

1 egg

2 green onions, sliced

Fresh cilantro, chopped, for garnish

1 Preheat the oven to 400°F.

2 Heat a nonstick skillet over high heat. Once hot, add 1 teaspoon of olive oil. Swirl to make a small circle of oil in the center of the pan. Add the shredded potato, and use a spatula to press down and flatten it. Dust the potato with half of the coriander and the cayenne pepper and salt. Drizzle the remaining teaspoon of olive oil over the potatoes.

3 Cook for about 4 minutes, until the bottom of the potato has browned, then use a spatula to flip. Season with the remaining coriander and another dash each of cayenne and salt. Continue cooking about 4 more minutes, until the bottom has turned golden brown. If the potatoes are browning too quickly, reduce the heat or remove from the heat completely.

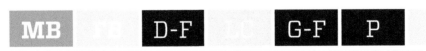

MB **D-F** **G-F** **P**

PER SERVING

Calories **324** Carbohydrates **25g** Fat **15g** Protein **24g**

4 Spoon the black beans onto the circle of potato, drizzle the salsa over the beans, and spread the Pulled Chicken on top. Make a well in the center of the chicken layer, and crack open the egg into the indent. Remove from the heat.

5 Transfer the skillet into the oven, and bake for 5 minutes, or until the egg is cooked to your preference. For a runnier egg yolk, decrease the cook time.

6 Garnish with the green onion and cilantro, and enjoy. You may also enjoy more salsa or some lime juice, hot sauce, or avocado slices (although these added toppings are not reflected in the recipe's nutritional breakdown).

Cooking tip: *If you do not have an ovenproof skillet, cook the hash browns on the stove until both sides are golden brown. Transfer the hash browns to a baking dish, assemble as described in the recipe, and bake for 5 minutes.*

Ingredient tip: *Store-bought hash browns can save you the time spent shredding the potato. Defrost according to package instructions before cooking.*

CHAPTER FOUR

CHICKEN & POULTRY

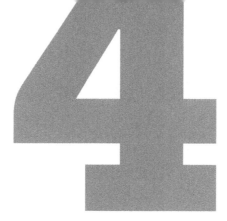

Yes, a fitness regimen paired with a diet that incorporates chicken and turkey has been proven to increase overall fat loss and improve muscle gains. But there's a false belief that this means bland, boring food. This chapter completely debunks that myth. Here, you will find a variety of recipes to keep your taste buds guessing.

All kinds of poultry provide a strong source of protein, B-vitamins, selenium, phosphorus, and essential fatty acids. Turkey has a slight nutritional advantage, but chicken tends to be more budget-friendly. To select the best cuts of poultry with the lowest total fat, saturated fat, and cholesterol, stick to white meat without skin, like skinless breast meat. If you can afford it, organic will reward you with more omega-3 fatty acids and fewer strains of dangerous antibiotic resistant bacteria. Taking it a step further, poultry that is "organic-plus" or "free range"—poultry that forages and pecks outdoors—is overall better quality meat with improved texture, taste, and nutrients.

Of course none of this makes a difference if it isn't prepared well! The cooking methods in the chapter ensure tender and moist meat that you will love eating on a daily basis. Each recipe has unique flavor combinations that make the meat taste great without adding a bunch of sugar and fat. This is healthy like you haven't tasted before!

MB Muscle Building **FB** Fat Burning **D-F** Dairy-Free **LC** Low Carb **G-F** Gluten-Free **P** Paleo **V** Vegan

TURKEY MEATBALLS
WITH MARINARA SAUCE

MAKES 30 MEATBALLS / PREP TIME: 30 MINUTES / COOK TIME: 20 MINUTES

Ideal for batch cooking

Low in calories, full of Italian flavor and the tiniest bit of heat—your taste buds
are in for a treat. These meatballs make a great appetizer, or try them on top
of spaghetti squash for a "spaghetti and meatball" dinner.

FOR THE TURKEY MEATBALLS

1 pound 99% fat-free ground turkey

2 egg whites

⅓ cup fresh basil, chopped

⅓ cup dried chopped onion

3 tablespoons nutritional yeast

2 tablespoons milled flaxseed

1 tablespoon minced garlic

1½ teaspoons Italian seasoning

1½ teaspoons dried parsley

1½ teaspoons crushed red pepper

FOR THE MARINARA DIPPING SAUCE

1 (14.5-ounce) can stewed tomatoes

1 (6-ounce) can no-salt-added
tomato paste

½ bell pepper, yellow or red, seeded
and chopped

¼ cup (about ½ medium)
chopped onion

1 tablespoon minced garlic

½ teaspoon salt

½ teaspoon freshly ground
black pepper

½ teaspoon dried oregano

½ teaspoon dried parsley

½ teaspoon dried rosemary

Extra-virgin olive oil spray

FB **D-F** **G-F** **P**

PER SERVING

Calories **78** Carbohydrates **3.2g** Fat **1.3g** Protein **13.2g** *3 w/o sauce*

Calories **117** Carbohydrates **11.9g** Fat **1.3g** Protein **14.4g** *3 w/ sauce*

TO MAKE THE TURKEY MEATBALLS

1 Preheat the oven to 400°F.

2 In a large bowl, mix well to combine the turkey, egg whites, basil, onion, nutritional yeast, flaxseed, garlic, Italian seasoning, parsley, and red pepper.

3 Using your hands, form approximately 30 meatballs each about 1 inch in diameter. Place the meatballs on a baking sheet lined with parchment paper or a silicone baking sheet.

4 Bake for 15 minutes. Flip the meatballs, and bake for another 3 to 5 minutes, until both sides have started to turn a slight golden brown.

5 Remove from the oven, and allow the meatballs to rest for 5 to 10 minutes.

TO MAKE THE MARINARA DIPPING SAUCE

1 While the meatballs rest, in a blender or food processor, blend the tomatoes, tomato paste, bell pepper, onion, garlic, salt, pepper, oregano, parsley, and rosemary until the mixture is smooth.

2 Spray a large pot with olive oil spray, add the marinara mixture, and simmer for 20 minutes, stirring frequently.

3 Serve the meatballs alone or with the marinara sauce on the side.

CRISPY CHICKEN
WITH SWEET MUSTARD DIP

**MAKES 5 (4-OUNCE) SERVINGS / PREP TIME: 15 MINUTES /
COOK TIME: 20 MINUTES**

This recipe has just as much crunch and flavor as fried chicken with only half the calories, healthy fats, and absolutely no gluten. If you've missed the crispy goodness of fried chicken, you're welcome!

FOR THE CRISPY CHICKEN

20 ounces boneless, skinless chicken
   breast, trimmed of fat and cut
   into strips
1½ cups crisp rice cereal
¼ cup dried minced onion
1 teaspoon salt
½ teaspoon ground red pepper
2 egg whites
1 tablespoon water
Extra-virgin olive oil spray

FOR THE SWEET MUSTARD DIP

1 tablespoon nonfat Greek yogurt
1 tablespoon Dijon mustard
1 teaspoon granulated stevia

TO MAKE THE CRISPY CHICKEN

1 Preheat the oven to 350°F.

2 Pat the chicken dry with a paper towel. Set aside.

3 In a sealed resealable bag, use a rolling pin or a can to crush the cereal into smaller pieces, being careful not to turn it into a powder. Pour the crushed cereal into a shallow bowl, add the onion, salt, and red pepper, and stir.

FB	D-F	LC	G-F	P

Calories **169** Carbohydrates **7g** Fat **3.7g** Protein **24g**
4 ounces

4 In a separate shallow bowl, stir well to combine the egg whites and water.

5 Dip a piece of the chicken into the egg whites, and allow any excess to drip back into the bowl. Dredge the chicken in the cereal mixture, pressing down to help it stick and making sure to cover all sides thoroughly.

6 Place the coated chicken on a baking sheet, and lightly spray each piece with the olive oil spray.

7 Bake for 8 to 10 minutes. Flip the chicken, spray lightly with more olive oil spray, and bake 8 to 10 minutes more.

TO MAKE THE SWEET MUSTARD DIP

1 While the chicken is baking, make the dipping sauce. In a small bowl, mix well to combine the yogurt, mustard, and stevia.

2 Serve the chicken fresh from the oven with the dipping sauce on the side.

PULLED CHICKEN

MAKES 12 (4-OUNCE) SERVINGS / PREP TIME: 10 MINUTES / COOK TIME: 6 HOURS

Ideal for batch cooking

By far one of the easiest things to cook, pulled chicken can be enjoyed in a multitude of ways. Try it in soups, salads, and tacos! An awesome way to change up your chicken and prep a ton of protein at once.

3 pounds skinless, boneless
   chicken breasts

1 large onion, chopped

1 bunch fresh cilantro, chopped

1½ cups salsa

¼ cup dried red peppers, lightly
   crushed (optional)

Time-saving tip: *This recipe freezes well, so feel free to pack it up in a storage container and store it away.*

1 In a slow cooker or a rice cooker with a slow cook setting, mix to combine the chicken, onion, cilantro, salsa, and red peppers (if using).

2 Cook for 4 to 6 hours on high.

3 Take the lid off the cooker, and stir the chicken. It should fall apart without much effort. If it is not breaking apart easily, set the cooker to high for another hour.

4 This is awesome by itself, or in tacos. Try it over black rice with a little avocado, salsa, and lime juice.

| FB | D-F | LC | G-F | P |

PER SERVING Calories **120** Carbohydrates **3g** Fat **1g** Protein **22g**

4 ounces

TURKEY SATAY SKEWERS

**MAKES 10 (4-OUNCE) SERVINGS /
PREP TIME: 10 MINS, PLUS 30 MINS TO MARINATE / COOK TIME: 15 MINS**

Ideal for batch cooking

If you are looking to add flavor to your turkey and spice up your meal without adding extra calories, these skewers are just the ticket. Try them with the Cucumber Salad (page 178).

½ cup rice vinegar

3 tablespoons freshly squeezed lime juice

3 tablespoons soy sauce (gluten-free, if desired) or liquid aminos

2 tablespoons yellow curry powder

4½ teaspoons garlic, minced

1½ teaspoons ground turmeric

1 teaspoon ground ginger

½ teaspoon ground cayenne pepper

½ teaspoon wasabi powder

2½ pounds turkey breast tenderloins, cubed

Cooking tip: *Turmeric and curry can stain bare skin, so wear gloves when handling, especially if you have acrylic nails.*

Serving tip: *Satay is typically served with a peanut dipping sauce. To make one, mix a little sriracha, stevia, and lime juice into a scoop of natural peanut butter.*

1 Preheat the grill to medium heat or the oven broiler to high, setting the rack about 8 inches from the heat.

2 In a small bowl, mix together the vinegar, lime juice, soy sauce, curry powder, garlic, turmeric, ginger, cayenne, and wasabi powder.

3 In a large resealable bag, combine the turkey with the marinade, seal the bag, and massage to ensure the turkey is well coated in the marinade to thoroughly coat. Refrigerate for at least 30 minutes, or longer if desired.

4 Thread the turkey pieces onto metal or bamboo skewers. For 4-ounce servings, divide evenly among 10 skewers.

5 Grill, or broil in the prepared pan, for 10 to 15 minutes, turning over once halfway through, and serve.

FB **D-F** **LC** **G-F**

PER SERVING

Calories **100** Carbohydrates **0g** Fat **1g** Protein **22g**

4 ounces

NOODLE-LESS TURKEY LASAGNA

MAKES 9 (3-BY-3-INCH) SERVINGS / PREP TIME: 40 MINUTES /
COOK TIME: 1 HOUR, 20 MINUTES / TOTAL TIME: 2 HOURS, 10 MINUTES

Ideal for batch cooking

Zucchini make a lovely—and healthy—alternative to wheat, or any other grain, pasta, especially if you're keeping calories and carbs in check, but crave that toothsome, cheesy deliciousness that lasagna offers by the forkful. My take on the Italian classic is packed with delicious authentic flavors and makes an amazing entrée, good for the whole family.

FOR THE MEAT SAUCE

1 pound 99% lean ground turkey

2 tablespoons minced garlic

1½ teaspoons freshly ground black pepper

Dash salt

1 large white onion, diced

1 large green bell pepper, diced

3 cups baby spinach, chopped

1 (15-ounce) can no-salt-added tomato sauce

1 (12-ounce) can no-salt-added tomato paste

2 tablespoons dried basil

1 tablespoon dried oregano

Ingredient tip: *Nutritional yeast is available online, in the bulk food section of many grocery stores, or in some health food aisles.*

FOR THE "NOODLES"

3 to 4 medium zucchini

1 small eggplant

Salt

FOR THE LASAGNA

1 (15-ounce) tub fat-free ricotta cheese

2 egg whites

2 tablespoons dried parsley

Extra-virgin olive oil spray

8 ounces fat-free mozzarella cheese, shredded

3 cups baby spinach

2 cups mushrooms, sliced

¼ cup nutritional yeast

MB   **G-F**

PER SERVING

Calories **202** Carbohydrates **20.7g** Fat **1.5g** Protein **31.2g**

1 square

TO MAKE THE MEAT SAUCE

1 Preheat the oven to 350°F.

2 Heat a large nonstick pot over medium-high heat. Add the ground turkey, garlic, pepper, and salt. Brown the turkey for about 5 minutes, stirring regularly.

3 Add the onion, bell pepper, and spinach, and cook for about 5 more minutes more, stirring regularly. At this point the meat should be completely cooked.

4 Add the tomato sauce, tomato paste, basil, and oregano, and stir. Bring the sauce to a boil, reduce the heat, and simmer for 20 minutes.

TO MAKE THE "NOODLES"

1 While the sauce simmers, slice the zucchini lengthwise into long, thin slices. The easiest way to do this is using a mandoline slicer. If you don't have one, you can also use the slicing blade of a box grater or a knife. Lightly salt the zucchini slices, and place in a large microwavable bowl. Cover with plastic wrap, poking one small slit in the cover, and microwave for 6 to 8 minutes, until tender. This will steam the zucchini. There is no need to add water before microwaving. After steaming, place the zucchini in a strainer to drain any liquid. Drier is better.

2 Slice, steam, and drain the eggplant using the same process.

TO ASSEMBLE THE LASAGNA

1 In a small bowl, mix together the ricotta, egg whites, and parsley until well blended.

2 Lightly spray a 9-by-13-inch pan with olive oil spray. Line up your ingredients, and begin to layer. Pour one-third of the meat sauce into the pan, spreading it over the bottom, top with one-third of the zucchini, then one-half of the ricotta mixture, half of the eggplant slices, and then half of the remaining meat sauce, followed by one-half of the mozzarella, all of the spinach, half of the remaining zucchini slices, the remaining ricotta mixture, the remaining eggplant slices, all of the mushrooms, the remaining meat sauce, the remaining zucchini, and the remaining mozzarella. Finish by sprinkling the nutritional yeast on top.

3 Place the pan on a foil-lined baking sheet for easy cleanup. Cover the pan with aluminum foil, and bake for 45 minutes.

4 Remove the foil, and cook for an additional 15 minutes.

5 Allow it to cool for at least 10 minutes.

6 Once the lasagna has cooled, slice it into 9 (3-by-3-inch) squares and serve.

TURKEY BURGER
ON AN EGGPLANT BUN

MAKES 7 PATTIES / PREP TIME: 10 MINUTES, PLUS 20 MINUTES TO SOAK /
COOK TIME: 20 MINUTES

Moist, full of flavor, and boosted with vitamins and healthy omega-3 fatty acids, these low-calorie burgers are a great way to satisfy your burger cravings. The melt-in-your mouth eggplant bun is hard to resist, but you can always go straight for the meat and enjoy the patty on its own.

FOR THE BUNS

2 tablespoons salt

2 large eggplants, sliced into
   1-inch-thick rounds

Extra-virgin olive oil spray

FOR THE BURGERS

1 pound 99% lean ground turkey

3 egg whites

½ cup (1 medium) diced bell pepper

¼ cup (1 medium) diced shallots

2 tablespoons milled flaxseed

1 tablespoon minced garlic

TO MAKE THE BUNS

1 Preheat the broiler.

2 Add the salt to a bowl large enough to fit the eggplant. Fill the bowl one-third full with water, and stir until the salt is completely dissolved. Add the eggplant to the bowl, and add more water if needed to cover it. It will float, so use a plate with something heavy on top to keep the eggplant slices submerged. Soak for 20 minutes.

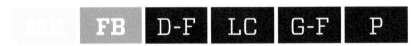

FB   D-F   LC   G-F   P

Calories **149** Carbohydrates **11.1g** Fat **5.6g** Protein **15.5g**

1 burger

3 Remove the eggplant from the salt water, and pat dry. Very lightly spray with the olive oil, and place on an oven rack or tray with vents. Allowing air to reach the bottom side will help the bottom dry out a bit faster.

4 Broil the eggplant slices 6 inches from the heat for about 5 minutes, until they are slightly browned. Flip them over, lightly oil the tops, and broil for another 5 minutes.

TO MAKE THE BURGERS

1 In a large bowl, mix to combine the turkey, egg whites, bell pepper, shallots, flaxseed, and garlic.

2 Use your hands to form 7 equal patties, and place them on a baking sheet. Broil about 8 inches from the heat until they are slightly brown, about 5 minutes. Flip over and broil for another 5 to 7 minutes.

3 Place a patty between two slices of eggplant. Serve with condiments of your choice, but keep in mind they will add calories to the dish. Try some nutritional yeast sprinkled on top for a cheesy taste, a little Dijon mustard, and some kale to add texture.

Cooking tip: *You could grill the burgers if you prefer, but typically they hold together better on the baking sheet.*

SPICY TURKEY STIR-FRY

SERVES 5 / PREP TIME: 5 MINUTES / COOK TIME: 20 MINUTES

Ideal for batch cooking

This filling and yummy—even with no noodles—variation to Mongolian barbecue is worth every bite. Pack it up in separate containers for five days of flavorful meals.

1 pound 99% fat-free ground turkey

1 medium onion, chopped

3 tablespoons minced garlic

Ground red pepper, as desired

1 large eggplant, chopped

3 to 5 tablespoons gluten-free Szechuan sauce

1 (8-ounce) can water chestnuts, drained

1 (8-ounce) can sliced bamboo, drained

1 (14-ounce) can sprouts, drained

1 bunch fresh cilantro, chopped

3 to 5 tablespoons soy sauce (gluten-free, if desired) or liquid aminos

1 In a large nonstick pot over medium-high heat, cook the turkey, onion, garlic, and red pepper (used to your preferred spiciness) until the turkey is lightly browned, about 5 minutes, stirring occasionally.

2 Add the eggplant and Szechuan sauce. If you are not a fan of spiciness, you could start with 3 tablespoons and add more if desired. Cook covered for about 5 minutes, stirring occasionally, until the eggplant is browned.

3 Add the water chestnuts, bamboo, sprouts, and cilantro. Add soy sauce to your preferred saltiness. Cook covered at a low simmer for about 8 more minutes, stirring occasionally.

4 Divide among five plates and serve.

FB **D-F** **G-F**

PER SERVING

Calories **175** Carbohydrates **16g** Fat **1.4g** Protein **24.2g**

HONEY-MUSHROOM CHICKEN

**MAKES 4 (4-OUNCE) SERVINGS / PREP TIME: 10 MINUTES /
COOK TIME: 15 MINUTES**

The sweet and savory sauce pushes your standard lean chicken breast and mushrooms dish to the yum-o side on the taste-o-meter. For a lower carb meal, try it with steamed broccoli, or have it over rice for a memorable post-workout meal.

1 pound skinless, boneless chicken breasts, sliced

2 garlic cloves, sliced

1 cup mushrooms, sliced

2 cups low-sodium chicken broth

2 tablespoons honey

1 tablespoon cornstarch

2 tablespoons water

Salt

Freshly ground black pepper

1 In a large nonstick pan over medium-high heat, brown the chicken breast, stirring frequently, for about 5 minutes.

2 Add the garlic and mushrooms, cover, and cook for about 5 minutes, until the mushrooms are tender.

3 Add the broth and honey, and stir. Bring to a simmer.

4 In a small bowl, mix the cornstarch and water. Stir the mixture into the pan. Simmer for about 5 more minutes, until the sauce has thickened.

5 Season with salt and pepper, divide among four bowls, and serve.

MB   **D-F**   **G-F**

PER SERVING

Calories **168** Carbohydrates **11.3g** Fat **1.8g** Protein **27.3g**

4 ounces

YOUR MOM'S HERB CHICKEN

**MAKES 6 (4-OUNCE) SERVINGS /
PREP TIME: 5 MINUTES, PLUS 2 HOURS TO MARINATE /
COOK TIME: 20 MINUTES / TOTAL TIME: 2 HOURS, 35 MINUTES**

Ideal for batch cooking

The herbal combination in this marinade will become your standard recipe for practically every large get-together you hold or go to—it's that much of a crowd pleaser. Grilling the chicken gives it that delectable smoky flavor we all crave in the summer. This protein-packed dish goes great with any salad or side.

1½ pound boneless, skinless
  chicken breast

2 tablespoons sesame oil

2 tablespoons balsamic vinegar

2 teaspoons dried basil

2 teaspoons dried oregano

2 teaspoons dried rosemary

1 teaspoon garlic powder

Dash salt

Dash freshly ground black pepper

1 In a large resealable bag, combine the chicken with the sesame oil, balsamic vinegar, basil, oregano, rosemary, garlic powder, salt, and pepper. Seal the bag and massage to ensure the chicken is well coated in the marinade. Refrigerate for at least 2 hours, or as long as overnight.

2 Preheat the grill or a large cast iron pan on the stove to medium-high heat.

3 Grill the chicken breast for 3 to 5 minutes per side, until browned on both sides. Turn the heat down to low, and continue to grill for up to 10 minutes more, until the chicken is cooked through and the center is no longer pink.

4 Transfer the chicken to a plate, and let it rest for 5 to 10 minutes before carving and serving.

FB	D-F	LC	G-F	P

PER SERVING

Calories **164** Carbohydrates **0.8g** Fat **6g** Protein **26g**

4 ounces

SPICY LATIN LIME CHICKEN

**MAKES 6 (4-OUNCE) SERVINGS / PREP TIME: 10 MINUTES /
COOK TIME: 20 MINUTES / TOTAL TIME: 40 MINUTES**

Ideal for batch cooking

This simple-to-make rub, full with a spicy kick, will rev up your metabolism and curb your hunger pangs.

FOR THE RUB

1 tablespoon ground cumin

1 tablespoon garlic powder

1½ teaspoons dried oregano

1 teaspoon ground coriander

1 teaspoon ground paprika

1 teaspoon freshly ground
   black pepper

1 teaspoon ground cayenne pepper

1 teaspoon ground cinnamon

FOR THE CHICKEN

24 ounces boneless, skinless chicken
   breast, trimmed of all fat

3 tablespoons freshly squeezed
   lime juice

Time-saving tip: *Make a big batch of the rub, and store it in an airtight container. Use as needed.*

Preheat the oven to 450°F.

TO MAKE THE RUB

In a shallow bowl, stir to mix the cumin, garlic powder, oregano, coriander, paprika, black pepper, cayenne pepper, and cinnamon.

TO PREPARE THE CHICKEN

1 Working one at a time, dredge the chicken breast in the spice blend, pressing one side in the rub, then the other, so that both are lightly coated. Place the chicken breasts in a single layer in a baking dish.

2 Bake for 15 to 18 minutes, until cooked through and no longer pink.

3 Remove the baking dish from the oven. Drizzle the lime juice evenly over the chicken breasts, and let rest for 5 to 10 minutes before carving.

| FB | D-F | LC | G-F | P |

PER SERVING

Calories **120** Carbohydrates **0g** Fat **1.5g** Protein **26g**

4 ounces

TURKEY STROGANOFF

SERVES 4 / PREP TIME: 5 MINUTES / COOK TIME: 20 MINUTES

With some healthy substitutes, this version of the famed Eastern European dish has much more protein and significantly less fat than its older sibling. Try pairing it with vegetables from the same region, like Sautéed Red Cabbage (page 197), or substitute noodles with Protein Mashed Potatoes (page 196).

1 pound 99% lean ground turkey

1 medium white onion, chopped

1 cup sliced mushrooms

8 teaspoons dried onion flakes

1½ teaspoons dried parsley

1 teaspoon onion powder

1 teaspoon ground turmeric

½ teaspoon celery seed

½ teaspoon salt, plus more
for seasoning

½ teaspoon granulated stevia

¼ teaspoon freshly ground black
pepper, plus more for seasoning

1 cup nonfat Greek yogurt

1 In a large, deep pan over medium-high heat, brown the ground turkey until almost cooked through, about 8 minutes.

2 Add the chopped onion and mushrooms, and stir in the onion flakes, parsley, onion powder, turmeric, celery seed, salt, stevia, and pepper. Cook for 10 minutes, stirring occasionally.

3 Remove from the heat, and stir in the yogurt until well-blended. Season with salt and pepper, and serve.

Serving tip: Traditionally, Stroganoff is served over egg noodles. Make this dish even healthier by serving it over brown rice, or serve it over mashed potatoes for a great post-workout meal (although these are not reflected in the recipe's nutritional breakdown).

FB   **G-F**

PER SERVING

Calories **174** Carbohydrates **9.5g** Fat **1g** Protein **33.5g**

WHOLE ROASTED CHICKEN

**MAKES 8 (4-OUNCE) SERVINGS / PREP TIME: 15 MINUTES /
COOK TIME: 1 HOUR, 10 MINUTES / TOTAL TIME: 1 HOUR, 35 MINUTES**

A beautifully roasted bird is a staple of the dinner table. Preparing the whole bird, rather than only the leanest cuts, does bring up the fat content, but enjoying a crisp-skinned, tender-fleshed chicken every so often won't kill your gains. Try this recipe next time you're roasting and you'll be rewarded with a moist bird infused with flavor.

1 (3½-pound) whole chicken, patted
   dry, giblets removed

2 teaspoons salt

Freshly ground black pepper

1 teaspoon dried rosemary

1 teaspoon ground sage

1 teaspoon dried thyme

¼ cup chopped celery

Serving tip: Nutritional information can vary based on white meat, dark meat, and whether you eat the skin. Assuming much of the weight is bones, a 3½-pound chicken should give you about 8 (4-ounce) servings.

1 Preheat the oven to 400°F.

2 Season the chicken inside and out with the salt and pepper. Place the chicken breast-side up in a roasting pan or Dutch oven. Dust the inside of the cavity with the rosemary, sage, and thyme, and stuff the cavity with celery. Roast for 1 hour.

3 Using a baster or large spoon, baste the chicken with the pan juices. Continue roasting for about 10 minutes longer, until the juices run clear when the thickest part of the thigh is pierced with a knife and the skin is golden and crisp.

4 Let the chicken rest for 10 minutes before carving and serving.

MB

D-F **LC** **G-F** **P**

PER SERVING

Calories **200** Carbohydrates **1.3g** Fat **12g** Protein **22.7g**

4 ounces

KUNG POW CHICKEN

SERVES 4 / PREP TIME: 15 MINUTES / COOK TIME: 15 MINUTES

Traditional Chinese style Kung Pow chicken is much healthier than what is served at your local restaurant. So why not make a more healthful variation with just as much flavor at home? Cashews add healthy fats and a nice nutty finish to this metabolism-boosting spicy dish. Serve with your favorite steamed vegetable, or over rice.

FOR THE SAUCE

2 tablespoons soy sauce (gluten-free, if desired) or liquid aminos

1 teaspoon honey

½ teaspoon apple cider vinegar

2 tablespoons water

1 teaspoon cornstarch

FOR THE MARINADE

2 teaspoons soy sauce (gluten-free, if desired) or liquid aminos

1 tablespoon rice vinegar

1 teaspoon cornstarch

FOR THE CHICKEN

1 pound boneless, skinless chicken breast, cut into 1-inch cubes

2 teaspoons sesame oil or coconut oil

¼ cup dried red chile peppers, seeded, stemmed, and halved

1 teaspoon peeled and minced fresh ginger

1 teaspoon minced garlic

¼ cup roasted cashews or peanuts

1 tablespoon chopped green onion

FB **D-F** **LC** **G-F**

PER SERVING

Calories **200** Carbohydrates **6.3g** Fat **7g** Protein **27.3g**

4 ounces

TO MAKE THE SAUCE

In a small bowl, mix together the soy sauce, honey, apple cider vinegar, water, and cornstarch. Set aside.

TO MAKE THE MARINADE

In a small bowl, stir together the soy sauce, rice vinegar, and cornstarch until the cornstarch has dissolved.

TO PREPARE THE CHICKEN

1 In a large bowl, pour the marinade over the chicken, and toss to coat.

2 In a large skillet over medium-high heat, heat 1 teaspoon of sesame oil. Add the chicken, and stir-fry for 5 minutes, until browned but not cooked through. Transfer to a plate and set aside.

3 Clean the skillet if needed, and heat the remaining 1 teaspoon of sesame oil over medium-high heat. Add the peppers, ginger, and garlic, and stir-fry for about 3 minutes, until the spices are aromatic.

4 Add the chicken, cashews, green onion, and sauce to the skillet, and stir until the meat is well coated. Stir-fry for about 5 more minutes, until the chicken is cooked through, and serve.

CHICKEN TORTILLA SOUP

SERVES 4 / PREP TIME: 10 MINUTES / COOK TIMES: 20 MINUTES

Ideal for pre-workout

The combination of chicken, beans, tortillas, and tomato-based ingredients provides a well-balanced meal of fast- and slow-digesting carbohydrates, protein, and fiber. It's just the mouthwatering meal you need to fuel your body through a tough workout. Note that I use Pulled Chicken (page 72) here, but you can use whatever cooked chicken you have on hand.

1 cup (1½ medium) chopped onion

2 teaspoons minced garlic

1 pound Pulled Chicken (page 72)

2 cups low-sodium chicken broth

1 (10-ounce) can enchilada sauce

1 cup (3 medium plum) chopped tomatoes

½ cup salsa

1 (15.5-ounce) can black beans, drained and rinsed

½ teaspoon ground cumin

¼ teaspoon ground paprika

¼ teaspoon freshly ground black pepper

Dash ground cayenne pepper

2 tablespoons freshly squeezed lime juice

4 (6-inch) corn tortillas, cut into small strips

¼ cup fresh cilantro, chopped

1 Heat a large nonstick pot over medium-high heat. Add the onion and garlic, and cook until the onions are softened, about 3 minutes.

2 Add the Pulled Chicken, press down, and cook undisturbed for about 2 minutes, until the bottom slightly browns.

3 Stir in the broth, enchilada sauce, tomatoes, salsa, black beans, cumin, paprika, black pepper, cayenne pepper, and lime juice. Bring to simmer, and cook for about 15 minutes, until heated through.

4 Divide among four bowls, garnish each with the tortilla strips and some cilantro, and serve. You may also enjoy a dollop of nonfat Greek yogurt or some avocado (although these toppings are not included in the nutritional information).

MB **D-F** **G-F**

PER SERVING

Calories **325** Carbohydrates **39.5g** Fat **3g** Protein **34.8g**

4 ounces

OVEN-ROASTED TURKEY BREAST

**MAKES 12 (4-OUNCE) SERVINGS / PREP TIME: 5 MINUTES /
COOK TIME: 1 HOUR / TOTAL TIME: 1 HOUR, 20 MINUTES**

Ideal for batch cooking

Why deal with the hassle of a whole bird when the only part we really want is the ultra-lean breasts? Whether it's the holidays or just another week of meal prep, pick up a turkey breast and roast away. You'll have enough turkey to feed an army.

1 (3-pound) boneless, skinless turkey breast half
1 tablespoon extra-virgin olive oil
1 tablespoon salt
1 teaspoon dried oregano
1 teaspoon dried rosemary
1 teaspoon dried thyme
½ teaspoon freshly ground black pepper
½ teaspoon garlic powder

Ingredient tip: *Look for turkey breasts in the chest coolers or in the butcher's display case of your local grocery store. One 3-pound half-breast should be plenty for a normal week. A whole breast would be more appropriate for a large family dinner.*

1 Preheat the oven to 375°F.

2 Rinse the turkey breast, and pat it dry. Place the breast in a baking dish. Using your hands, massage the olive oil and salt onto all sides of the breast. Sprinkle the oregano, rosemary, thyme, pepper, and garlic powder evenly over the turkey breast.

3 Roast for about 1 hour, until the juices run clear when pierced with a fork. Start checking after 50 minutes of roasting, and continue checking every 10 minutes until done.

4 When cooked, remove the turkey from the oven and cover loosely with foil. Rest the turkey for 15 minutes before carving.

5 Slice the breast crosswise into slices against the grain and serve.

FB	D-F	LC	G-F	P

PER SERVING

Calories **131** Carbohydrates **0g** Fat **2.2g** Protein **24.3g**

4 ounces

SUPERFOOD CHICKEN SOUP

**MAKES 8 (2-CUP) SERVINGS / PREP TIME: 10 MINUTES /
COOK TIME: 1 HOUR, 25 MINUTES**

Ideal for batch cooking

Hearty, full of flavor, plus all the goodness your body needs in one bowl, this
recipe will definitely leave you satisfied. Superfoods like spinach, kale, broccoli, and Brussels sprouts in combination with the protein boost of lean
chicken breast supercharge your body with nutrients.

2 cups (3 medium) chopped
  white onion

1 cup (2 stalks) chopped celery

1½ teaspoons minced garlic

24 ounces skinless, boneless chicken
  breasts, cut into ½-inch cubes

4 cups low-sodium chicken broth

1 (15-ounce) can no-salt-added
  tomato sauce

3 cups tightly packed baby spinach

3 cups chopped kale

2 cups broccoli, chopped

2 cups Brussels sprouts, quartered

2 cups (3 medium) chopped carrot

2 cups (about ¾ pound) green
  beans, chopped

1 teaspoon freshly ground black
  pepper

1 teaspoon red pepper flakes

½ teaspoon dried basil

½ teaspoon celery seed

½ teaspoon ground allspice

½ teaspoon ground ginger

Pinch ground cinnamon

3 to 4 cups water

FB **D-F** **G-F** **P**

PER SERVING

Calories **179** Carbohydrates **18.4g** Fat **1.8g** Protein **23.5g**

2 cups

1 Heat a large nonstick pot over medium-high heat. Add the onion, celery, and garlic, and cook for about 3 minutes.

2 Add the chicken, and stir. Cook for about 5 more minutes.

3 Stir in the broth and tomato sauce, and bring to a simmer. Add the spinach, kale, broccoli, Brussels sprouts, carrot, green beans, black pepper, red pepper flakes, basil, celery seed, allspice, ginger, and cinnamon. Bring to a simmer, and cook for 15 minutes.

4 Add 3 to 4 cups of water, depending on desired thickness. Continue to simmer for 45 minutes to 1 hour more, until the vegetables are tender, and serve.

Ingredient tip: *This is an everything-but-the-kitchen-sink type of recipe. You can use fresh or frozen veggies. Feel free to throw in any other nutritious vegetables you have lying around.*

Time-saving tip: *This soup stores well. Pack it up into airtight storage containers and store for a week. If it thickens in the fridge, add a little more water before warming it up.*

PEANUT CHICKEN

**MAKES 4 (4-OUNCE) SERVINGS / PREP TIME: 10 MINUTES /
COOK TIME: 15 MINUTES**

If you are trying to lean out, this recipe is the one for you. No added fat or
sugar keeps the calories and carbs low, but thanks to the incredible flavor,
you would have never guessed it. The marinade is full of peanut goodness,
which adds a touch more protein to the ultra-lean chicken breasts.

FOR THE PEANUT SAUCE

4 tablespoons light-roast defatted
   peanut flour

1 tablespoon granulated stevia

3 tablespoons soy sauce (gluten-free,
   if desired) or liquid aminos

3 teaspoons rice vinegar

¼ teaspoon ground cayenne pepper

FOR THE CHICKEN AND VEGETABLES

2 cups broccoli florets

1 tablespoon water

Extra-virgin olive oil spray

3 tablespoons minced garlic

4½ teaspoons chopped fresh ginger

24 ounces boneless, skinless chicken
   breasts, cut into 2-inch strips

¾ cup chopped green onion

2 tablespoons water, as needed

FB	D-F	LC	G-F

PER SERVING

Calories **143** Carbohydrates **3.4g** Fat **2.5g** Protein **28.7g**

4 ounces

TO MAKE THE PEANUT SAUCE

In a large bowl, mix to combine the peanut flour, stevia, soy sauce, vinegar, and cayenne, and stir until smooth. Set aside.

TO MAKE THE CHICKEN AND VEGETABLES

1 Place the broccoli florets and water in a medium microwave-safe bowl. Cover with plastic wrap, and cut a small slit to vent steam. Microwave on high for 5 minutes, or until tender. Drain off any water from the bowl.

2 Heat a large skillet over medium-high heat, and lightly coat with olive oil spray. Add the garlic and ginger, and cook for 1 minute.

3 Add the chicken, and cook about 7 minutes, until cooked through. Add the green onion, and cook for 1 minute more.

4 Transfer the chicken to the bowl with the peanut sauce, add the steamed broccoli, and toss to coat with the sauce. If the sauce is too thick, add the water 1 teaspoon at a time, tossing after each addition, to desired consistency.

5 Divide the chicken and broccoli among four plates, and serve.

CHICKEN AND VEGGIE ONE-DISH WONDER

SERVES 6 / PREP TIME: 10 MINUTES / COOK TIME: 30 MINUTES

Ideal for pre-workout

This one-dish meal covers all the bases: protein from lean chicken breast, carbs from nutrient-packed sweet potato, a colorful mix of fibrous veggies, and a light layer of healthy olive oil. Aromatic herbs, onion, and citrus complement each other nicely for a simple yet savory flavor you are going to love.

24 ounces boneless, skinless chicken breast, cut into 1-inch cubes

2 tablespoon balsamic vinegar

Extra-virgin olive oil spray

18 ounces Brussels sprouts, quartered

18 ounces sweet potato (about 3 to 4 medium), cut into 1-inch cubes

18 ounces zucchini (about 4 medium), cut into half rounds

6 ounces red onion (about 1 ½ to 2 medium), cut into bite-size chunks

4 garlic cloves, sliced

¼ cup orange juice or freshly squeezed lemon juice

1 teaspoon dried basil

1 teaspoon dried crushed bay leaf

1 teaspoon dried rosemary

1 teaspoon freshly ground black pepper

Salt

| MB | D-F | G-F | P |

PER SERVING

Calories **275** Carbohydrates **27.8g** Fat **4g** Protein **30.7g**

(4 ounces chicken, 3 ounces sweet potatoes, a mixture of remaining veggies)

1 Preheat the oven to 400°F.

2 In a medium bowl, drizzle the cubed chicken breast with the balsamic vinegar. Toss to coat. Set aside to marinate while you prepare the vegetables.

3 Lightly coat the bottom of a large baking dish with olive oil spray. Add the Brussels sprouts, sweet potato, zucchini, onion, and garlic, mix together, and spread into a single layer (if possible).

4 Spread the marinated chicken over the bed of vegetables, and pour any remaining balsamic over all.

5 Spray the contents of the baking dish very lightly with the olive oil spray.

6 Drizzle the orange juice over all, and sprinkle with the basil, crushed bay leaf, rosemary, and pepper, and season with salt.

7 Bake for about 30 minutes, until the sweet potatoes are tender and the chicken is cooked through, and serve.

GRILLED LEMON CHICKEN

**MAKES 6 (4-OUNCE) SERVINGS /
PREP TIME: 5 MINUTES / COOK TIME: 40 MINUTES**

Ideal for batch cooking

In a hurry and not wanting to wait for the meat to marinate? This is a convenient recipe full of fat-burning citrus and vitamin C that needs no planning ahead. Grilling the chicken and adding the dressing later makes this lean protein moist and tender, as if you had marinated it overnight. If you are feeling fancy, you can kick things up a notch with grilled lemon slices.

FOR THE DRESSING

2 tablespoons freshly squeezed
   lemon juice

2 tablespoons fresh oregano,
   finely chopped

1 tablespoon lemon zest

1 tablespoon garlic, minced

1 tablespoon extra-virgin olive oil

½ teaspoon salt

½ teaspoon freshly ground
   black pepper

FOR THE CHICKEN

1 ½ pounds boneless, skinless
   chicken breasts

Salt

Freshly ground black pepper

2 lemons, cut crosswise into
   ¼-inch-thick slices

FB **D-F** **LC** **G-F** **P**

PER SERVING

Calories **141** Carbohydrates **0.5g** Fat **3.9g** Protein **26g**

4 ounces

Preheat both sides of the grill to medium-high heat.

TO MAKE THE DRESSING

In a small bowl, whisk together the lemon juice, oregano, lemon zest, garlic, olive oil, salt, and pepper.

TO PREPARE THE CHICKEN

1 Sprinkle both sides of the chicken breasts with salt and pepper. Turn off one grill side, and leave the other burning. Place the chicken breasts over the burner that is off. Close the cover, and grill for 30 minutes, turning the chicken once after 15 minutes, until the chicken is no longer pink in the center.

2 Remove the chicken from the grill, and place it in a large bowl. Pour the dressing over the chicken, and toss to coat. Leave the chicken to rest in the dressing for 10 minutes.

3 While the chicken is resting, grill the lemons uncovered over the lit burner for about 3 minutes per side, until grill marks appear.

4 Divide the chicken breasts among plates, garnish with the grilled lemon slices, and serve.

Cooking tip: *If you prefer a sweeter dressing, try adding 1 tablespoon stevia or honey. Remember to add the calories to the nutritional breakdown here.*

TURKEY LETTUCE WRAPS

MAKES 8 WRAPS / PREP TIME: 10 MINUTES / COOK TIME: 10 MINUTES

Full of protein and packed with flavor, this revisited favorite is also lower in fat and sugars than the restaurant version. Prep-to-table is super quick, and the wraps can be had as appetizers, a snack, or a light meal.

FOR THE SAUCE

⅓ cup soy sauce (gluten-free, if desired) or liquid aminos

3 tablespoons apple cider vinegar or rice vinegar

2 tablespoons honey

1 tablespoon Dijon mustard

1 tablespoon sriracha

½ teaspoon sesame oil

3 to 4½ teaspoons granulated stevia (optional)

FOR THE FILLING

1 teaspoon avocado oil, olive oil, or sesame oil

1 pound 99% lean ground turkey

2½ teaspoons minced garlic

⅛ teaspoon ground ginger

8 ounces white mushrooms, chopped

4 green onions, chopped

1 (6-ounce) can water chestnuts, drained and chopped

FOR THE WRAPS

8 large iceberg lettuce leaves

1 cup bean sprouts

½ cup shredded carrot (about 1½ medium)

½ cup fresh cilantro, chopped

FB	D-F	LC	G-F

PER SERVING

Calories **100** Carbohydrates **7.5g** Fat **1.5g** Protein **15g**

1 wrap

TO MAKE THE SAUCE

In a small bowl, whisk together the soy sauce, vinegar, honey, mustard, sriracha, and sesame oil. Taste the sauce. If you prefer it sweeter, add the stevia. Set the sauce aside.

TO MAKE THE FILLING

1 In a large pan over medium-high heat, heat the oil. Add the turkey, garlic, and ginger, and cook for about 5 minutes, until no longer pink.

2 Add the mushrooms, green onions, and water chestnuts, and cook for about 5 minutes, until the mushrooms are tender.

3 Pour the prepared sauce evenly over the turkey mixture, stir, and cook for 1 minute more, until heated through. Remove from the heat.

TO ASSEMBLE THE WRAPS

1 Place a lettuce leaf on a plate. Spoon one-eighth (about 2 ounces) of the turkey mixture into the lettuce cup. Repeat with the remaining lettuce leaves and turkey mixture.

2 Garnish each wrap with sprouts, carrot and cilantro, and serve.

MANDARIN CHICKEN

MAKES 4 (4-OUNCE) SERVINGS / PREP TIME: 10 MINS / COOK TIME: 10 MINS

Ideal for post-workout

This inspired dish is light without the usual breading or grease. Sweet mandarin orange sections infuse the sauce with their citrusy-sweet flavor while keeping the chicken tender. Healthy carbs from the fruit and honey fuel your muscles after a hard workout. Serve with your favorite steamed veggies, or over rice.

1 (15-ounce) can no-sugar-added mandarin oranges

1 pound boneless, skinless chicken breast, cut into 1-inch cubes

Salt

2 tablespoons honey

2 tablespoons freshly squeezed lemon juice

1 tablespoon soy sauce (gluten-free, if desired) or liquid aminos, plus more for garnish (optional)

1½ teaspoons ground ginger

1½ teaspoons cornstarch

Extra-virgin olive oil spray

1 teaspoon orange zest

1⁄2 teaspoon crushed red pepper (optional), plus more for garnish

1 Open the can of mandarin oranges, and drain the liquid into a large bowl. Transfer ¼ cup of the liquid into a small bowl, and set aside. Season the chicken with salt, and add it to the mandarin liquid in the large bowl. Toss to coat and set aside.

2 Add the honey, lemon juice, soy sauce, ginger, and cornstarch to the reserved ¼ cup of mandarin liquid, and whisk until the cornstarch dissolves. Set aside.

PER SERVING   Calories **231** Carbohydrates **27.5g** Fat **1.5g** Protein **27g**   *4 ounces*

3 Heat a large nonstick pan over medium heat, and lightly coat with the olive oil spray. Add the chicken and any remaining marinade to the pan, and cook for about 5 minutes, until all sides of the chicken are brown.

4 Stir in the honey mixture, and bring to a gentle simmer. Simmer for about 4 minutes, until the sauce has thickened and the chicken is cooked through. Add in the orange zest, crushed red pepper (if using), and mandarin oranges. Cook for about 1 minute, until the mandarin oranges are heated through. Remove from the heat.

5 Divide among four plates, garnish with more soy sauce, or crushed red pepper if you prefer, and serve.

CURRY CHICKEN
WITH CAULIFLOWER "RICE"

SERVES 4 / PREP TIME: 10 MINUTES / COOK TIME: 25 MINUTES

If you've been looking for a reduced-fat, no-added-sugar curry to soothe a craving, your search is over. This chef-worthy dish has everything good from the dish that is its inspiration and none of the bad stuff. Tender chicken? Check! Curried coconutty flavors? Check! Rice to sop up the soupy yummi-ness? Check! The "rice" is the best part: riced cauliflower replaces white rice, reducing carbs and sneaking in a muscle-building cruciferous veggie.

1 teaspoon coconut oil

2 tablespoons curry powder, plus more for seasoning

1 cup chopped white onion (about 1½)

1 tablespoon minced ginger

1½ teaspoons minced garlic

3 cups (a little less than 1 medium) 1-inch-cubed eggplant

1 tablespoon lemongrass paste

1 (13.5-ounce) can reduced-fat unsweetened coconut milk

1 pound boneless, skinless chicken breast, cut into 1-inch cubes

Salt (optional)

1 large head cauliflower

1 lime, quartered

Fresh cilantro, chopped, for garnish

1 In a large pot over medium heat, heat the coconut oil. Add the curry powder and cook, stirring, until fragrant, about 1 minute.

2 Add the onion, ginger, and garlic, and cook, stirring often, reducing the heat if necessary to prevent browning, until softened, about 4 minutes.

3 Increase the heat to medium, and add the eggplant and lemongrass paste. Cook, stirring occasionally, for about 5 minutes, until the vegetables are just beginning to soften.

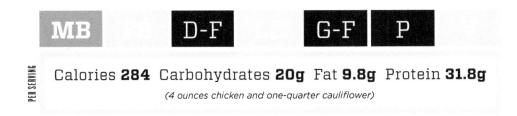

MB	D-F	G-F	P

PER SERVING

Calories **284**   Carbohydrates **20g**   Fat **9.8g**   Protein **31.8g**

(4 ounces chicken and one-quarter cauliflower)

4 Add the coconut milk and enough water to cover the eggplant, and bring to a simmer. Add the chicken, and simmer very gently for about 10 minutes, until the chicken is cooked through. Season with salt or curry powder for extra flavor.

5 While the curry is cooking, prepare the cauliflower. To rice the cauliflower, remove the stem and chop the head into small florets. Using a food processor, blender, or grater, process the cauliflower into pieces the size of rice. Put the riced cauliflower in a microwave-safe bowl, cover, and microwave on high for 3 minutes, or until the cauliflower is tender. A larger head of cauliflower will need more time to cook.

6 Divide the cauliflower rice and curry among four plates, squeeze one lime quarter over each, sprinkle with cilantro, and serve.

Ingredient tip: *Purchase canned coconut milk at your local grocery store in the ethnic food aisle. It is different from the coconut milk beverage that comes in cartons and sits next to the almond and soy milk.*

Cooking tip: *If you are using a processor or blender, don't add too many florets at a time or it may take a while, and you may end up with mushy patches. Some grocery stores now carry bags of riced cauliflower, so check your local store; you may be in luck! If you prefer, however, just steam small florets of cauliflower to go with the curry. Spaghetti squash makes an exceptional cauliflower rice substitute.*

ORANGE-INFUSED CHAI CHICKEN

**MAKES 2 (4-OUNCE) SERVINGS / PREP TIME: 5 MINUTES /
COOK TIME: 30 MINUTES / TOTAL TIME: 45 MINUTES**

A light dusting of chai seeps into the chicken as it bakes on a bed of orange slices. The result is a savory mixture of fat-burning orange citrus with all the earthy blend of clove, cinnamon, and ginger in the chai tea that will help keep your blood sugar stable. Using a covered dish steams the chicken breast to a moist and tender finish. This pairs perfectly with a salad, or baked sweet potatoes.

1 orange
1 (8-ounce) chicken breast
2 tablespoons water
1 chai tea bag
Salt

1 Preheat the oven to 350°F.

2 Cut the orange in half. From the center of the orange, cut three rounds about ¼ inch thick from one of the halves. Lay the rounds in a row in a small baking dish with a cover.

3 Place the chicken breast over the orange rounds, and squeeze the juice from the remaining orange half over the chicken breast. Add the water, pouring around, but not on, the chicken.

4 Carefully tear open the packet of chai, and lightly dust the top of the chicken breast with some of its contents. You do not have to use all of the contents. More will give a stronger taste. Season with salt.

5 Cover the dish, and bake for 30 minutes.

6 Remove from the oven, and let it rest, covered, for 10 minutes before serving.

Time-saving tip: To make more servings at once, line the bottom of the entire dish with orange rounds, cover it in a layer of chicken breast, and use enough tea packets to lightly dust all of them.

| FB | D-F | LC | G-F | P |

PER SERVING

Calories **137** Carbohydrates **4g** Fat **2g** Protein **26g**

4 ounces

TOM KHA GAI

SERVES 4 / PREP TIME: 5 MINUTES / COOK TIME: 20 MINUTES

A rich and creamy coconut milk soup that is a favorite at Thai restaurants. My version simplifies it a bit, with ingredients you probably already have at home, and slims it down to decrease overall calories and added sugars. What's left is all the amazing flavors that make it a joy to eat chicken and healthful coconut fats.

1 teaspoon coconut oil or extra-virgin olive oil

1 pound boneless, skinless chicken breast, cut into thin strips

1 teaspoon minced garlic

1 teaspoon salt

1 cup sliced mushrooms

2 tablespoons lemongrass paste

Pinch ground cayenne pepper

1 (13.5-ounce) can reduced-fat unsweetened coconut milk

2 cups water

⅓ cup fresh cilantro, chopped, plus more for garnish

¼ cup freshly squeezed lime juice, plus more for garnish

Ingredient tip: *Purchase canned coconut milk at your local grocery store in the ethnic food aisle. It is different from the coconut milk beverage that comes in cartons and sits next to the almond and soy milk.*

1 In a large nonstick saucepan over medium-high heat, heat the coconut oil. Add the chicken, garlic, and salt, and cook for about 5 minutes, until the chicken browns.

2 Stir in the mushrooms and lemongrass paste, and cook for about 5 minutes, until the mushrooms are tender.

3 Stir in the cayenne, coconut milk, water, cilantro, and lime juice. Bring to a simmer, and continue cooking for 10 more minutes.

4 Divide among four bowls and serve. If you prefer, garnish with more cilantro and lime juice.

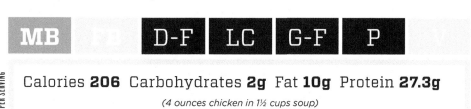

MB **D-F** **LC** **G-F** **P**

PER SERVING

Calories **206** Carbohydrates **2g** Fat **10g** Protein **27.3g**

(4 ounces chicken in 1½ cups soup)

ROASTED GARLIC–STUFFED ITALIAN BAKED CHICKEN

**MAKES 8 (4-OUNCE) SERVINGS / PREP TIME: 10 MINUTES /
COOK TIME: 30 MINUTES / TOTAL TIME: 50 MINUTES**

What's not to love about roasted garlic? Stuffing chicken with melt-in-your-mouth roasted garlic, topping it with ultra-healthy nutritional yeast that imbues the chicken with that nutty parmesan flavor, and topping it all with marinara and mozzarella! Who needs an Italian restaurant when you have this? Pair with your favorite green veggies or salad greens for a low-carb and low-fat meal.

1 yellow onion, sliced into rings

2 pounds boneless, skinless chicken breasts

16 roasted garlic cloves (see ingredient tip), halved lengthwise

Salt

Freshly ground black pepper

Pinch crushed red pepper, or more if desired

¼ cup nutritional yeast

1 (15-ounce) can no-salt-added crushed tomatoes

1 tablespoon Italian seasoning

1 fresh basil sprig, chopped

½ cup nonfat mozzarella, shredded (optional)

1 Preheat the oven to 375°F.

2 In the bottom of a large baking pan with a cover, place the onion slices in a thin layer.

3 Fillet each chicken breast horizontally and open as you would a book. Spread the roasted garlic evenly among the breasts, and close them back up so that the cloves are layered inside each breast.

FB **LC** **G-F**

PER SERVING

Calories **172** Carbohydrates **8.1g** Fat **1.5g** Protein **30.8g**

4 ounces

4 Place the chicken over the onion in the pan, and season each breast with salt, black pepper, and crushed red pepper. Spread the nutritional yeast evenly over the breasts, and then spoon the crushed tomatoes over all, gently spreading it with the back of a spoon to evenly coat each breast. Sprinkle the Italian seasoning, basil, and mozzarella (if using) on top.

5 Cover and bake the chicken for 20 minutes. Remove the cover, and bake for 10 minutes more, until the center is no longer pink.

6 Remove from the oven and let rest for 10 minutes before serving.

Ingredient tips: Nutritional yeast is available online, in the bulk food section of many grocery stores, or in some health food aisles.

You could roast your own garlic from fresh cloves, or buy it already roasted at the store. To roast it yourself, peel most of the outer layer from each head of garlic, leaving the cloves intact. Chop enough off of the end of each head to expose the cut cloves inside. Drizzle with olive oil, wrap in aluminum foil, and bake in a 400°F oven for about 40 minutes, until golden and the cloves in the center pierce easily with a knife.

CABBAGE ROLLS

**MAKES 8 TO 10 CABBAGE ROLLS / PREP TIME: 30 MINUTES /
COOK TIME: 2 HOURS**

Tender cabbage leaves hug a delectable filling of protein-rich ground turkey and spinach, with the added cheesy richness of nutritional yeast. These are great as a snack, appetizer, or main dish.

1 head napa cabbage

1 cup water

2 pounds 99% lean ground turkey

1 teaspoon freshly ground
  black pepper

½ teaspoon salt

½ teaspoon dried basil

1 cup (about 1½ medium) diced
  yellow onion

1 teaspoon garlic, minced

4 cups fresh baby spinach, chopped

⅓ cup nutritional yeast

1 (8-ounce) can crushed tomatoes

1 (4-ounce) can tomato sauce

Serving tip: This recipe should make 8 to 10 rolls, depending on how big the leaves are. For the nutritional information here, it is assumed that each roll has one-eighth of the meat mixture, approximately 4 ounces of turkey meat.

1 Preheat the oven to 350°F.

2 Using a knife, remove the cabbage's core. Place the cabbage in a microwave-safe bowl. Add the water, and cover with plastic wrap, making a slit to vent. Microwave on high for 12 minutes, or until the leaves are tender and peel away easily.

3 While the cabbage is steaming, heat a medium nonstick skillet over medium-high heat, and add the ground turkey. Sprinkle the turkey with the pepper, salt, and basil. Cook until the turkey has browned, about 8 minutes. Drain off any liquid.

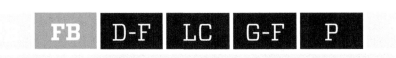

| FB | D-F | LC | G-F | P |

PER SERVING

Calories **153** Carbohydrates **7.5g** Fat **1g** Protein **29.4g**

(1 cabbage roll with 4 ounces filling)

4 Add the onion and garlic, and cook for about 5 minutes more, until the onion is translucent.

5 Add the spinach, and cook for about 2 minutes, until the spinach is wilted. Stir in the nutritional yeast, remove from heat, and set aside to cool.

6 In a small bowl, mix together the crushed tomatoes and tomato sauce. Spread half of the mixture in the bottom of a 9-by-13-inch baking dish, and reserve the other half.

7 When the cabbage is cool enough to handle, gently peel off 10 whole leaves one by one.

8 Lay one leaf down cup-side up with the stem facing you. Place ⅓ cup of the turkey mixture in the center of the leaf. Fold the stem end over the mixture, then fold the sides toward the center, then roll the package away from you. Place each roll, stem-side down, in the baking dish. Repeat with the remaining cabbage leaves and turkey filling. When all the cabbage rolls are done, pour the remaining tomato mixture evenly over the top.

9 Cover the dish with foil, bake for 90 minutes, and serve.

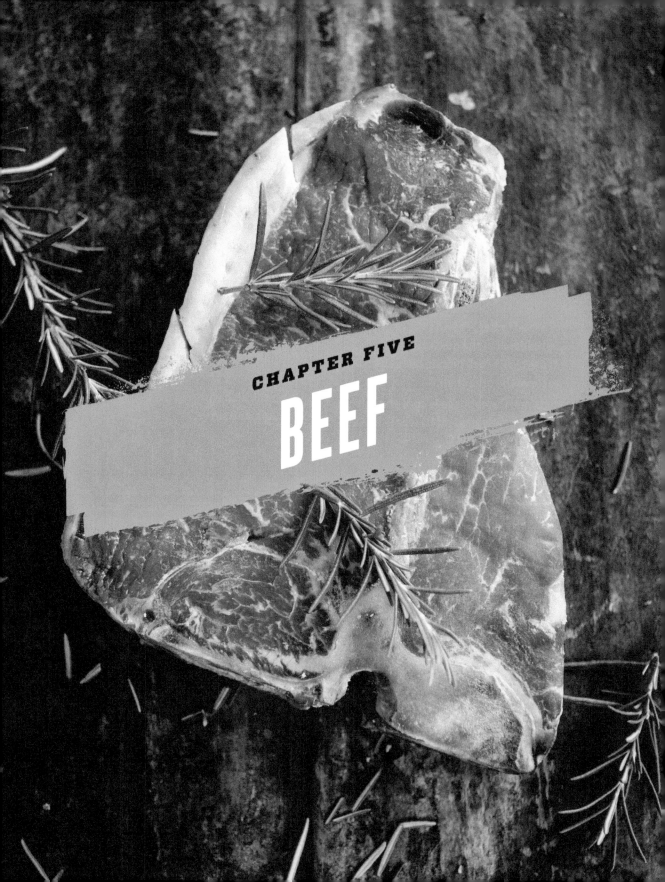

CHAPTER FIVE

BEEF

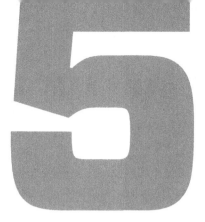

Here's the secret to adding beef—a source of protein, zinc, iron, and B-vitamins our bodies need to build some serious muscle—to your diet successfully: know your cuts. You want to avoid artery-clogging fats, so select the leanest cuts of beef, preferably from grass-fed cattle because they offer far greater benefits. Ironically, the leanest cuts of beef tend to be more affordable because, except for the fitness-minded, everyone else wants tender cuts marbled with fat. Beef eye round is by far the leanest, followed by top round, bottom, round, top sirloin, and chuck shoulder, each with only 4 to 5 grams or less of total fat per serving. The trick is to cook them using the right technique so they end up just as juicy as the fattier cuts of beef. The recipes in this chapter will help you navigate through all the details, and show you great ways to eat extra-lean ground beef, grill up some T-bones, or slow cook a round roast. Remember, beef is great!

MB Muscle Building **FB** Fat Burning **D-F** Dairy-Free **LC** Low Carb **G-F** Gluten-Free **P** Paleo **V** Vegan

THE BEST BEEF RUB

MAKES ABOUT 5 TABLESPOONS / PREP TIME: 5 MINUTES

Ideal for batch cooking

A combination guaranteed to rev up your metabolism, this is a great rub to keep on hand. An easy way to add deep and complex flavors to your favorite cut without any of the calories.

2 tablespoons finely ground coffee

4½ teaspoons granulated garlic

4½ teaspoons salt

1 heaping teaspoon freshly ground black pepper

¼ teaspoon ground cayenne pepper

¼ teaspoon ground cinnamon

¼ teaspoon ground cloves

1 In a small bowl, mix well to combine the coffee, garlic, salt, black pepper, cayenne pepper, cinnamon, and cloves.

2 Store in a sealed storage container.

Cooking tip: *If you have the time, allow meat with the rub to rest refrigerated anywhere from 2 hours to overnight for best results.*

Time-saving tip: *Prepare in bulk by multiplying all ingredients by the desired amount. Store the unused portion in an airtight container for later use.*

FB **D-F** **LC** **G-F** **P**

PER SERVING

Calories **0** Carbohydrates **0g** Fat **0g** Protein **0g**

GRILLED MARINATED STEAK

**MAKES 4 (4-OUNCE) SERVINGS /
PREP TIME: 10 MINUTES, PLUS 4 HOURS TO MARINATE /
COOK TIME: 15 MINUTES / TOTAL TIME: 4 HOURS, 35 MINUTES**

Ideal for batch cooking

This is a great marinade to enhance the naturally delicious flavors of your steak, without covering them up. Top sirloin steaks are more tender than the other round cuts, making them the ultimate choice for grilling.

1 tablespoon extra-virgin olive oil

1 teaspoon garlic, minced

4½ teaspoons apple cider vinegar

4½ teaspoons balsamic vinegar

4½ teaspoons soy sauce (gluten-free, if desired) or liquid aminos

1½ teaspoons yellow mustard

⅛ teaspoon ground cloves

Freshly ground black pepper

16 ounces top sirloin steaks, trimmed of all fat (trimmed tip steak or ball tip steak)

Cooking tip: *Take the steaks out of the refrigerator at least 20 minutes prior to cooking them. This allows them to adjust to room temperature so they cook more evenly.*

1 In a small bowl, mix the olive oil, garlic, apple cider vinegar, balsamic, soy sauce, mustard, cloves, and pepper until well combined.

2 Carefully transfer the marinade to a 1-gallon resealable bag, and add the steaks. Massage the bag to ensure the steaks are well coated.

3 Refrigerate for at least 4 hours, preferably overnight.

4 Preheat the grill or a large cast iron pan on the stove to high heat.

5 Grill for 7 to 15 minutes, depending on the thickness of the steak and your preferred doneness.

6 Let the steak rest for 5 to 10 minutes before carving against the grain and serving.

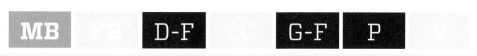

MB **D-F** **G-F** **P**

PER SERVING

Calories:**170** Carbohydrates **0g** Fat **8.3g** Protein **24g**

4 ounces

GARLIC AND ROSEMARY GRILLED T-BONES

**MAKES 5 TO 7 (4-OUNCE) SERVINGS / PREP TIME: 10 MINUTES /
COOK TIME: 15 MINUTES / TOTAL TIME: 35 MINUTES**

While T-bones are a fattier cut of beef, enjoying them sparingly shouldn't be a problem. A classic paste made with rosemary, garlic, and olive oil is an easy way to add flavor to an already delicious choice of meat that takes very well to grilling.

Leaves of 3 fresh rosemary sprigs,
  finely chopped
1½ teaspoons garlic, minced
¼ teaspoon crushed red pepper flakes
1 teaspoon extra-virgin olive oil
2 (20-ounce) T-bone steaks,
  room temperature
Salt (optional)

Cooking tip: Taking the steaks out of the refrigerator at least 20 minutes prior to cooking allows them to adjust to room temperature so they cook more evenly.

Ingredient tips: The inedible bone and tendons account for about 29 percent of the steak's weight. Keep this in mind when trying to prepare your edible ounces.

1 In a small bowl, stir the rosemary, garlic, crushed red pepper, and olive oil into a loose paste.

2 Spread the mixture evenly over the steaks, and season with salt (if using).

3 Preheat the grill to medium-high heat. Ensure the grill is clean.

4 Place the steaks on the hottest part of the grill, and quickly sear both sides until they are brown, less than 2 minutes per side.

5 Move the steaks to a cooler part of the grill, and cook to desired doneness, about 5 to 6 more minutes per side.

6 Remove the steaks from the grill, and let rest for 5 to 10 minutes.

7 Cut the steak off the bone, slice across the grain, and serve.

| MB | | D-F | LC | G-F | P | |

PER SERVING

Calories **223** Carbohydrates **0g** Fat **10.1g** Protein **30.9g**

4 ounces

EYE ROUND STEAK

MAKES 2 (4-OUNCE) SERVINGS / PREP TIME: 5 MINUTES / COOK TIME: 30 MINUTES / TOTAL TIME: 40 MINUTES

The quick-sear-and-bake method is a surefire way to lock in juices and make sure an ultra-lean steak won't come out chewy, dry, or tough.

1 (8-ounce) boneless eye of
  round steak
2 pinches salt (optional)
1 teaspoon coconut oil
Freshly ground black pepper

Cooking tips: Take the steaks out of the refrigerator at least 20 minutes prior to cooking them. This allows them to adjust to room temperature so they cook more evenly.

If you prepare multiple servings at once that you plan to reheat later, leave the steak rare. When you warm it up later, it will not get overcooked.

Eye of round is very lean. Carving it thinly against the grain will make it more tender.

1 Preheat the oven to 300°F.

2 Line a baking sheet with nonstick aluminum foil.

3 Pat the steak surfaces dry, and sprinkle each side with a pinch of salt (if using).

4 In a large skillet over high heat, heat the coconut oil until you see gentle smoke lifting off of the surface.

5 Using tongs, place the steak in the skillet, and sear for 1 minute on each side.

6 Place the steaks in the prepared baking sheet, and bake for 20 to 30 minutes, checking often to make sure the steak does not overcook. This steak is best served rare to medium rare.

7 Remove from the oven and let rest for 5 minutes.

8 Carve against the grain in thin slices and serve.

FB **D-F** **LC** **G-F** **P**

PER SERVING

Calories:**150** Carbohydrates **0g** Fat **6g** Protein **24g**

4 ounces

STEAK AND VEGETABLE SOUP

**MAKES 10 (2-CUP) SERVINGS / PREP TIME: 30 MINUTES /
COOK TIME: 1 HOUR, 45 MINUTES**

Ideal for batch cooking • Ideal for post-workout

A hearty and flavorful soup stuffed with steak and veggies. The added russet potatoes provide some fast-absorbing carbohydrates to refuel your body after a tough workout.

1½ teaspoons extra-virgin olive oil, divided

¼ pound boneless eye of round, trimmed of all fat and cut into bite-size cubes

3 celery ribs, chopped

1 large yellow onion, chopped

4 cups tomato juice or V8

3½ cups low-sodium beef broth

3 carrots, chopped

2 russet potatoes, chopped

2 (14-ounce) cans no-salt-added diced tomatoes

2 small dried bay leaves

1 cup frozen corn

2 teaspoons garlic powder

1 cup frozen peas

2 teaspoons hot sauce

Cooking tip: If your pot can't hold more than 20 cups easily, cut the recipe in half.

1 Warm a large pot over medium-high heat. Heat ¾ teaspoon of olive oil, and add the beef. Cook until all sides are brown, about 5 minutes. Remove from the pot, and set aside.

2 Add the remaining ¾ teaspoon of olive oil to the pot, followed by the celery and onion, and cook for 10 minutes.

3 Add the browned beef, tomato juice, broth, carrots, potatoes, diced tomatoes, bay leaves, corn, and garlic to the pot, and stir to combine. Bring to a boil. Reduce the heat, and simmer uncovered for 1 hour.

4 Add the peas and hot sauce to the soup, cover, and simmer for about 30 minutes longer.

5 Remove the bay leaves, ladle into bowls, and serve.

MB   **D-F**   **G-F**

PER SERVING

Calories **181** Carbohydrates **18.5g** Fat **5.2g** Protein **15.8g**

2 cups

15-MINUTE BEEF CHILI

MAKES 5 (2-CUP) SERVINGS / PREP TIME: 10 MINUTES / COOK TIME: 15 MINUTES

Ideal for batch cooking • Ideal for pre-workout

Even when your cupboards look bare, you can pull together this quick one-pot meal that barely needs any prep. Not only is it no-fuss, this chili also offers a great balance of protein (with ground beef and two kinds of beans) and carbohydrates.

1 pound extra-lean ground beef

½ medium green bell pepper, seeded and diced

½ cup chopped red onion (about 1 medium)

½ teaspoon minced garlic

1 (16-ounce) can red beans, drained and rinsed

1 (16-ounce) can red kidney beans, drained and rinsed

1 (28-ounce) can chopped no-salt-added stewed tomatoes

1 tablespoon chili powder

1 tablespoon ground cumin

¼ teaspoon dried oregano

½ cup salsa

Ingredient tip: *If you are trying to lean out, substitute ground turkey for the ground beef.*

1 Heat a large pot over medium-high heat. Add the ground beef, bell pepper, and onion, and cook for about 5 minutes, until browned. Drain off any grease, if necessary.

2 Add the garlic, red beans, kidney beans, tomatoes, chili powder, cumin, oregano, and salsa, and cook for 7 to 10 minutes more, until heated through, stirring frequently.

3 Ladle into bowls and serve.

Serving tip: *Try topping with a dollop of Greek yogurt in place of sour cream, a few diced chives, or a spoonful of salsa. Just remember to change the nutritional information accordingly.*

MB **D-F** **G-F**

PER SERVING

Calories **236** Carbohydrates **27.4g** Fat **3.8g** Protein **23.6g**

2 cups

SLOPPY JOES

MAKES 5 (1-CUP) SERVINGS / PREP TIME: 5 MINUTES / COOK TIME: 15 MINUTES

Ideal for post-workout

This hot-sweet take on a ubiquitous everyday quick meal is sure to become a favorite. That touch of honey and stevia, paired with the jalapeño and cinnamon, melds with the other ingredients into a satisfying post-workout meal. Serve over a baked russet or sweet potato to carb up after a tough workout— or you can go for a lighter option and simply serve on a lettuce leaf.

1 pound extra-lean ground beef

1 yellow onion, diced

1 (15-ounce) can no-salt-added
   tomato sauce

2 tablespoons no-salt-added
   tomato paste

1 tablespoon apple cider vinegar

1 tablespoon honey

1 tablespoon granulated stevia,
   plus more if desired

1 tablespoon soy sauce (gluten-free,
   if desired) or liquid aminos

1 teaspoon mustard powder

Pinch ground cinnamon

¼ teaspoon freshly ground black pepper

1 medium red bell pepper, seeded
   and diced

1 medium green bell pepper, seeded
   and diced

2 teaspoons minced garlic

1 jalapeño, seeded and minced (optional)

1 Heat a large nonstick skillet over medium-high heat. Add the beef and onions, and cook for about 5 minutes, until brown. Drain off any grease, if necessary.

2 While the beef is browning, in a small bowl, stir to combine the tomato sauce, tomato paste, apple cider vinegar, honey, stevia, soy sauce, mustard powder, cinnamon, and pepper until well blended. Set the sauce aside.

3 Add the red pepper, green pepper, garlic, and jalapeño (if using) to the beef, and cook for about 5 minutes more, stirring often.

4 Stir in the prepared sauce. Reduce the heat, simmer for about 5 minutes, and serve.

MB　　**D-F**　　**G-F**

PER SERVING

Calories **193** Carbohydrates **18.4g** Fat **4.8g** Protein **20g**

1 cup

APPLE AND OATS MEATLOAF

**MAKES 4 SLICES / PREP TIME: 10 MINUTES / COOK TIME: 1 HOUR /
TOTAL TIME: 1 HOUR, 25 MINUTES**

You will love the taste, texture, and extra health benefits the apples and oats add to this home-cooked comfort food. It's classic meatloaf, made better.

1 pound extra-lean ground beef

1 cup no-salt-added tomato juice or tomato sauce

1 cup (about 1½ medium) apple, peeled, cored, and finely chopped

¾ cup whole rolled oats

1 egg, lightly beaten

¼ cup (about ½ medium) white onion, chopped

1½ teaspoons dried parsley

½ teaspoon salt (optional)

¼ teaspoon freshly ground black pepper

⅛ teaspoon ground allspice

⅛ teaspoon mustard powder

1 Preheat the oven to 350°F.

2 In a large bowl, mix lightly but thoroughly to combine the beef, tomato juice, apple, oats, egg, onion, parsley, salt (if using), pepper, allspice, and mustard powder. Do not overmix or you will end up with a tough meatloaf. Press the mixture into an 8-by-4-inch loaf pan, and bake for 1 hour.

3 Remove from the oven and let sit for about 15 minutes.

4 Slice into four even pieces and serve. If there are any leftovers, this loaf tastes even better the next day.

MB   **D-F**   **G-F**   **P**

PER SERVING | Calories **234** Carbohydrates **17.5g** Fat **7g** Protein **26g** | 1 slice

POT ROAST

MAKES 12 (4-OUNCE) SERVINGS / PREP TIME: 15 MINUTES /
COOK TIME: 3 HOURS, 10 MINUTES

Ideal for batch cooking

Chuck roast is a very affordable cut of meat that provides protein nearly as lean as top sirloin and round roast. It is a great choice for this tender pot roast. When it's ready, the little cubes of meat will melt in your mouth.

1 tablespoon extra-virgin olive oil, divided

2 medium onions, peeled and quartered

6 carrots, unpeeled, cut into 2-inch pieces

1 (3-pound) chuck roast, trimmed of all fat

Freshly ground black pepper

About 4 cups low-sodium beef broth, divided

Leaves of 3 fresh rosemary sprigs

Leaves of 3 fresh thyme sprigs

1 Preheat the oven to 275°F.

2 In a large pot or Dutch oven over medium-high heat, heat 1½ teaspoons of olive oil. Add the onions and carrots, and cook for 5 to 7 minutes, until lightly brown. Remove the onions and carrots from the pot, and set aside.

3 Generously season the chuck roast with pepper. Add the remaining 1½ teaspoons of olive oil to the pot, and increase the heat to high. Place the roast in the pot, and sear it for 1 minute on each side, until brown. Transfer the roast to a plate.

4 With the burner still on high, add 1 cup of broth to the pot and deglaze, using a spoon to scrape up any browned bits from the bottom. Place the roast back in the pot, and add enough stock to come halfway up the meat. Add the onions and carrots, spreading them around the roast. Loosely sprinkle the rosemary and thyme on top of the roast.

5 Cover the pot, transfer to the oven, and roast for 3 hours.

6 The roast is ready to serve when the meat is tender and falls apart easily.

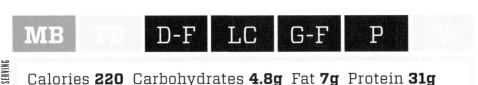

PER SERVING

MB D-F LC G-F P

Calories **220** Carbohydrates **4.8g** Fat **7g** Protein **31g**

≈ 4 ounces

SLOW COOKER BEEF STEW

MAKES 8 (2-CUP) SERVINGS / PREP TIME: 20 MINUTES / COOK TIME: 6 HOURS

Ideal for batch cooking

This is a simple "set it and forget it" dish that is great to make when you want to come home to a soul-satisfying meal. Affordable, lean chuck roast tossed with russet potatoes and carrots help nourish you post-workout. Try making it in bulk so you can have it on hand when you get home after a long day.

1 (2-pound) chuck roast, trimmed of all fat and cut into bite-size pieces

2 cups low-sodium beef broth

1 (15-ounce) can no-salt-added diced tomatoes

2 cups baby carrots

2 russet potatoes, peeled and cut into 1-inch cubes

1 large onion, finely chopped

2 celery ribs, sliced

1 tablespoons soy sauce (gluten-free, if desired) or liquid aminos

1 tablespoon apple cider vinegar

1 tablespoon dried parsley

1 teaspoon dried oregano

1 teaspoon freshly ground black pepper

1½ teaspoons minced garlic

¼ cup water

¼ cup cornstarch

1 In the slow cooker, stir to combine the roast, broth, tomatoes, carrots, potatoes, onion, celery, soy sauce, apple cider vinegar, parsley, oregano, pepper, and garlic. Cook on high for 6 hours.

2 About 30 minutes before it is done cooking, in a small bowl, mix the water and cornstarch together, and pour the mixture into the slow cooker. Mix well, and cook for the remaining 30 minutes.

3 Skim the top of your stew to remove and discard as much of the fat as you can, ladle the stew into bowls, and serve.

Cooking tip: *Most rice cookers have a slow cooker setting.*

The great thing about slow cooking is you don't have to watch it. If you leave it in a little too long, the timer will shut it down to a lower heat. The vegetables may be a bit overcooked, but it will still taste great.

MB **D-F** **G-F**

PER SERVING

Calories **269** Carbohydrates **18.8g** Fat **8.1g** Protein **28.9g**

2 cups

HIGH-HEAT EYE OF ROUND ROAST

**MAKES 12 (4-OUNCE) SERVINGS / PREP TIME: 5 MINUTES /
COOK TIME: 2 HOURS, 50 MINUTES / TOTAL TIME: 3 HOURS, 10 MINUTES**

Ideal for batch cooking

Eye of round is the leanest cut. This simple but flavorful technique results in a tender texture without adding any sugar or fat. Perfection.

1 (3-pound) eye of round roast, trimmed of all fat
1 teaspoon salt
1 teaspoon freshly ground black pepper
2 teaspoons minced garlic
½ teaspoon dried thyme
½ teaspoon dried rosemary

1 Preheat the oven to 500°F.

2 Season the roast with the salt, pepper, garlic, thyme, and rosemary. Place in a foil-lined roasting pan or baking dish for easy cleanup. Do not cover or add water.

3 Place the roast in the oven, and immediately reduce the temperature to 475°F. From now until the end of cooking, do *not* open the oven door until the roast is completely done. Doing so will allow precious heat to escape, and the roast may not cook all the way through.

4 After 21 minutes (larger roasts will need more time; allow for 7 minutes more per extra pound), turn off the oven and allow the meat to continue roasting for 2½ hours.

5 Remove the roast from the oven, and let it rest for 15 minutes.

6 Carve into thin slices against the grain and serve.

	FB	D-F	LC	G-F	P	

PER SERVING

Calories **185** Carbohydrates **0** Fat **5g** Protein **34g**

4 ounces

PUERTO RICAN BISTEC ENCEBOLLAO

MAKES 8 (4-OUNCE) SERVINGS /
PREP TIME: 15 MINUTES, PLUS 4 HOURS TO MARINATE / COOK TIME: 40 MINUTES
Ideal for batch cooking

Puerto Rico's take on steak and onions is a simple one-skillet recipe with complex delicious flavors. Serve with rice and cilantro as garnish for a complete meal.

2 pounds top sirloin steak, thinly sliced against the grain

2 large white onions, sliced into rings

1½ cups low-sodium beef broth or water

½ cup apple cider vinegar

¼ cup (about 2 limes) freshly squeezed lime juice

2 tablespoons extra-virgin olive oil

2 tablespoons minced garlic

1 teaspoon salt

½ teaspoon ground coriander

½ teaspoon ground cumin

½ teaspoon ground paprika

⅛ teaspoon dried oregano

1 Put the steak, onions, broth, apple cider vinegar, lime juice, olive oil, garlic, salt, coriander, cumin, paprika, and oregano in a large resealable bag. Massage to ensure the meat is well coated. Marinate in the refrigerator for at least 4 hours.

2 Pour the contents of the bag into a large, deep skillet over medium-high heat, and bring to a boil. Reduce the heat to low, cover, and simmer for about 40 minutes, stirring occasionally, until the beef is tender.

3 Serve.

MB **D-F** **LC** **G-F** **P**

PER SERVING

Calories **259** Carbohydrates **5.8g** Fat **24.6g** Protein **24.2g**

4 ounces

SALISBURY STEAK
WITH MUSHROOM AND ONION GRAVY

**MAKES 8 (4-OUNCE) SERVINGS / PREP TIME: 20 MINUTES /
COOK TIME: 20 MINUTES**

Ideal for batch cooking

Garlic, onion, and mushrooms add flavor and nutrients to this affordable
meal. This dish embraces the hint of earthiness and toothsome quality of
mushrooms. Try it with creminis, or use whatever you have on hand.

FOR THE HAMBURGER STEAKS

2 pounds extra-lean ground beef

1 egg

1 teaspoon minced garlic

½ yellow onion, minced

1 teaspoon garlic powder

1 teaspoon onion powder

1 teaspoon freshly ground black
    pepper

1 teaspoon dried thyme

FOR THE GRAVY

1 tablespoon extra-virgin olive oil

½ yellow onion, minced

½ teaspoon minced garlic

1 (8-ounce) package mushrooms,
    sliced

1 cup beef broth, divided

1 tablespoon cornstarch

1 teaspoon freshly ground black
    pepper

½ teaspoon salt

½ teaspoon garlic powder

½ teaspoon onion powder

MB **D-F** **LC** **G-F**

PER SERVING

Calories **170** Carbohydrates **3g** Fat **6.9g** Protein **24.9g**

4 ounces

TO MAKE THE HAMBURGER STEAKS

1 In a large bowl, mix to combine the beef, egg, garlic, onion, garlic powder, onion powder, pepper, and thyme. Using your hands, form eight oval patties of equal size.

2 In a large nonstick skillet over medium-high heat or on a grill, cook the patties for 3 to 5 minutes per side. Cooking time will vary depending on thickness and desired doneness.

TO MAKE THE GRAVY

1 In a large skillet over medium-high, heat the olive oil. Add the onion, garlic, and mushrooms and cook for about 7 minutes, until the onion becomes translucent and slightly browned, stirring frequently.

2 In a small bowl, stir together 2 tablespoons of broth and the cornstarch. When the cornstarch has dissolved, stir in the remaining broth, and add the liquid to the skillet. Stir until slightly thickened, and then add the pepper, salt, garlic powder, and onion powder. Cook for an additional 5 minutes, stirring frequently. Remove from the heat.

3 Place one hamburger steak on each plate, top with a generous scoop of mushroom-onion gravy, and serve.

PERSIAN BEEF KEBABS

**MAKES 12 (4-OUNCE) SKEWERS /
PREP TIME: 20 MINUTES, PLUS 6 HOURS TO MARINATE / COOK TIME: 10 MINUTES**

Ideal for batch cooking

You will love the taste and texture of these delicious skewers after the enzymes in the Greek yogurt work their magic and tenderize the lean cut of protein into a soft and tender kebab. Topped with the hot and tangy dressing, the kebabs are simply perfect—served with grilled vegetables, or on top of cauliflower "couscous."

FOR THE MARINADE

½ cup nonfat Greek yogurt

1 tablespoon apple cider vinegar

1 tablespoon freshly squeezed
   lemon juice

1 tablespoon minced garlic

2 teaspoons hot sauce

1 teaspoon ground cumin

1 teaspoon salt

¼ teaspoon freshly ground
   black pepper

FOR THE KEBABS

3 pounds bottom round steak, cut into
   1-inch cubes

Coconut or extra-virgin olive oil, for
   oiling the grill

1 large yellow onion, chopped slightly
   larger than the beef cubes

TO MAKE THE MARINADE

1 In a large bowl, whisk together the yogurt, apple cider vinegar, lemon juice, garlic, hot sauce, cumin, salt, and pepper.

2 Reserve half the marinade in a separate bowl. Cover and refrigerate until later.

FB **LC** **G-F**

PER SERVING

Calories **152** Carbohydrates **1.2g** Fat **4g** Protein **25g**
(1 skewer with 4 ounces beef)

TO MAKE THE KEBABS

1 Add the beef cubes to a large resealable bag. Add the remaining marinade, and massage the bag to ensure all the beef is well coated. Marinate in the refrigerator for at least 6 hours and up to overnight.

2 Preheat the grill to medium-high. Ensure the grill is clean. Lightly oil the grill. Alternatively, preheat the oven broiler to high, set the rack about 8 inches from the heat, and line a broiler pan with aluminum foil.

3 Thread the beef cubes and onion pieces onto 12 skewers, alternating the beef and onion. Grill for 3 to 4 minutes on each side for medium-rare.

4 Place the kebabs on a serving platter, and drizzle with the reserved marinade, or remove the skewers, place the meat in your meal prep containers, and drizzle with the reserved marinade.

Time-saving tip: *Prepare the skewers based on your desired serving size. For 4-ounce servings, divide the beef and onions evenly among 12 skewers. For 6-ounce servings, divide the beef and onions evenly among 8 skewers.*

STUFFED BELL PEPPERS

**MAKES 4 STUFFED PEPPERS / PREP TIME: 20 MINUTES /
COOK TIME: 40 MINUTES**

Bell peppers are chock-full of vitamins C, A, and B, minerals (folate, potassium, manganese), and antioxidants. They are a true font of nutritional goodness. Stuffed with lean ground beef and kale, you can bet this is what superheroes dine on.

FOR THE STUFFING

1½ teaspoons extra-virgin olive oil

2 cups shredded kale

⅓ cup (about 1 medium) finely chopped white onion

1½ teaspoons minced garlic

¼ cup (about 2 stalks) finely chopped green onion

2 tablespoons minced green bell pepper (use any flesh clinging to removed tops)

1 pound extra-lean ground beef

1 cup canned diced tomatoes

1 tablespoon dried parsley

1½ teaspoons Italian seasoning

1 teaspoon seasoning salt or seasoning blend

FOR THE STUFFED PEPPERS

4 large green bell peppers, seeds and tops removed

¼ cup of liquid reserved from canned diced tomatoes

¼ cup tomato paste

¼ teaspoon minced garlic

¼ teaspoon dried oregano

¼ teaspoon dried basil

¼ cup low-fat mozzarella cheese, shredded, divided

MB

G-F

PER SERVING

Calories **316** Carbohydrates **17.8g** Fat **14.8g** Protein **28.8g**

1 stuffed pepper

Preheat the oven to 375 °F.

TO MAKE THE STUFFING

1 In a large pan over medium-high, heat the olive oil. Add the kale, onion, and garlic, and cook until the onion softens, about 5 minutes, stirring frequently.

2 Add the green onion and bell pepper, and cook for 5 minutes more, stirring frequently. Remove the mixture from the pan, and set aside.

3 Add the ground beef to the pan, and cook for 5 to 7 minutes, until cooked through.

4 Add the kale, onion, and pepper mixture back into the pan along with the tomatoes, parsley, Italian seasoning, and seasoning salt, and mix well. Cook for about 5 minutes, stirring frequently, until warmed through. Remove from the heat.

TO MAKE THE STUFFED PEPPERS

1 Fill each of the hollow green peppers with one-quarter of the stuffing. Pour the reserved tomato liquid into a baking dish, and place the peppers in the dish on the tomato liquid.

2 In a small bowl, stir together the tomato paste, garlic, oregano, and basil. Top each stuffed pepper with one-quarter of the mixture, and sprinkle each pepper with 1 tablespoon of the mozzarella.

3 Bake in the oven for 20 minutes, or until the cheese is golden brown, and serve.

Ingredient tip: *If you are trying to lean out, you can substitute ground turkey for beef and omit the mozzarella.*

ORANGE BEEF

SERVES 4 / PREP TIME: 20 MINUTES, PLUS 1 HOUR TO MARINATE / COOK TIME: 10 MINUTES

Ideal for batch cooking

Tangy from the citrus juice and zest, sweet from the honey, spicy from hot chili paste—a combo that will boost your metabolism and help you burn fat. The flavors are close-your-eyes-and-sigh delicious. This pairs well with Forbidden Fried Rice (page 198).

1 pound top sirloin steak, cut against the gain into thin strips

¼ cup orange juice

¼ cup rice vinegar

2 tablespoons soy sauce (gluten-free, if desired) or liquid aminos

1 tablespoon hot chili paste

1 tablespoon granulated stevia

1 teaspoon minced garlic

¼ cup water

1 teaspoon cornstarch

Extra-virgin olive oil spray

1 bunch green onions, sliced, white and green parts separated

2 tablespoons grated orange zest

Salt

Freshly ground black pepper

1 Put the beef, orange juice, rice vinegar, soy sauce, hot chili paste, stevia, and garlic in a resealable bag. Massage the bag to ensure the meat is well coated. Marinate in the refrigerator for at least 1 hour.

2 Over a small bowl, use scissors to cut one of the bottom corners off the resealable bag, and squeeze all the marinade from the bag into the bowl. Add the water and cornstarch to the marinade, and whisk until the cornstarch is dissolved. Set aside.

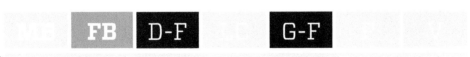

FB   D-F   G-F

PER SERVING

Calories **245** Carbohydrates **11g** Fat **12g** Protein **23.3g**

4 ounces

3 Heat a large nonstick skillet over high heat, and lightly coat with olive oil spray. Add the beef, and cook for 2 minutes, stirring occasionally.

4 Stir in the white parts of the green onions and the orange zest, and cook for 1 minute.

5 Stir in the marinade and the remaining green onions, season with salt and pepper, and cook for 3 to 5 minutes, until the beef is cooked through and the sauce has thickened.

6 Divide among four plates and serve.

Ingredient tip: *If you don't have hot chili paste on hand, you can substitute crushed red peppers or sriracha.*

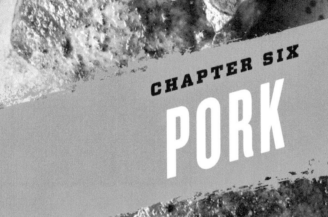

CHAPTER SIX

PORK

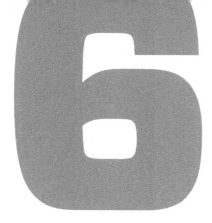

Tired of choking down chicken breasts to get shredded? I've got good news for you. Studies have shown that regularly incorporating lean pork into your diet improves body fat composition just as effectively as chicken. Pork also contains more B-vitamins than beef or chicken, helping improve metabolism and energy production, and providing a great dietary source of iron and zinc. To get the most protein per calorie, these recipes focus on leaner cuts, like pork tenderloin, pork loin, and pork shoulder trimmed of any excess fat. As an added bonus, these cuts of pork can be very affordable, especially if you buy them in larger quantities, an awesome option for prepping your meals in bulk. Best of all, pork is just as versatile and easy to cook as chicken. It's delicious in everything, from Hawaiian-Style Pork and Pineapple Skewers, to simple Almond-Crusted Pork Cutlets. Move those chicken breasts to the back burner, and get ready to enjoy pork like you never have before.

MB Muscle Building **FB** Fat Burning **D-F** Dairy-Free **LC** Low Carb **G-F** Gluten-Free **P** Paleo **V** Vegan

MEXICAN CARNITAS

**MAKES 14 (4-OUNCE) SERVINGS / PREP TIME: 15 MINUTES /
COOK TIME: 5 HOURS / TOTAL TIME: 5 HOURS, 25 MINUTES**

Ideal for batch cooking

Carnitas are a delicious choice for lean protein and are perfect for bulk preparations. Their melt-in-your-mouth moist, juicy tenderness and their crispy edges make them an easy reach, day after day. They are delicious over rice, in tacos, on salads—the possibilities are endless.

1 (4-pound) skinless, boneless
  pork shoulder
1 tablespoon extra-virgin olive oil
4½ teaspoons salt
1 tablespoon dried oregano
2 teaspoons ground cumin
1 teaspoon freshly ground
  black pepper
1 large yellow onion (about 6 ounces),
  coarsely chopped
1 jalapeño pepper, seeded and
  chopped
2 teaspoons minced garlic
1 tablespoon finely grated orange zest,
  plus ¾ cup freshly squeezed orange
  juice (from about 2 oranges)
Extra-virgin olive oil spray

1 On a work surface, using a sharp knife, trim the pork of all but a ¼-inch layer of fat. In a large bowl, rub the pork all over with the olive oil. Sprinkle with the salt, oregano, cumin, and pepper, and rub to coat.

2 Place the pork in a slow cooker or a rice cooker with a slow cook setting with the fat side facing up. Sprinkle with the onion, jalapeño, and garlic.

3 Squeeze the juice from the oranges over the pork, and sprinkle the grated peel over the top.

MB		D-F	LC	G-F	P

PER SERVING

Calories **205** Carbohydrates **0.5g** Fat **11g** Protein **26g**

4 ounces

4 Cook on high for about 5 hours. The pork is done when it is tender and breaks apart with very little effort.

5 Transfer the pork from the slow cooker to a platter, let rest for 5 to 10 minutes, and then shred the pork using two forks. Skim off and discard the fat from the juices. Refrigerate the juices for when reheating pork.

6 Heat a large pan over high heat for 1 minute, and lightly coat with the olive oil spray. Add the amount of shredded pork you're ready to serve, press down with a spatula, and cook until the bottom side is golden brown. Leave the top side as is, and serve.

To freeze: *Pack the pulled pork in airtight containers, portioning 1 week's worth of meal prep in each container (this will allow you to defrost only what is needed when the time comes). Distribute the juices from the slow cooker evenly among the containers.*

Serving tip: *If you are reheating, add the shredded pork to the pan as in step 6. Stir to warm through. If it dries out in the pan, pour a little of the juices on top.*

MUSTARD-CRUSTED PORK TENDERLOIN

MAKES 6 (4-OUNCE) SERVINGS /
PREP TIME: 10 MINUTES, PLUS 10 MINUTES TO MARINATE /
COOK TIME: 25 MINUTES / TOTAL TIME: 45 MINUTES

The herb-and-mustard crust adds tremendous taste without tons of calories to this excellent source of lean protein. The aroma while the tenderloin is in the oven will make your mouth water—guaranteed! A simple recipe with a 5-star experience.

1 (1½-pound) pork tenderloin, trimmed of excess fat

½ cup balsamic vinegar

¼ cup brown or Dijon mustard

¼ cup minced garlic

¼ cup dried minced onion

2 tablespoons freshly ground black pepper

2 tablespoons chopped fresh rosemary

2 tablespoons fresh thyme leaves

½ teaspoon chopped fresh dill weed

1 Preheat the oven to 425°F.

2 Place the pork tenderloin in a large bowl. Add the balsamic vinegar, and turn to coat. Let it marinate at room temperature for 10 minutes.

3 Meanwhile, in a medium bowl, mix the mustard with the garlic, dried onion, pepper, rosemary, thyme, and dill. It will form a very thick paste.

4 Place the tenderloin on a foil-lined baking sheet, and pour the balsamic on top.

5 Using your hands, press the paste in an even layer onto the top and sides of the tenderloin. Roast for 20 to 25 minutes.

6 Remove from the oven and let rest on the baking sheet for 10 minutes.

7 Transfer to a cutting board, slice the tenderloin against the grain into six equal pieces, and serve.

FB | **LC** | **G-F** | **P**

PER SERVING

Calories **151** Carbohydrates **8g** Fat **2.5g** Protein **24g**

4 ounces

ASIAN PORK ROAST

MAKES 12 (4-OUNCE) SERVINGS /
PREP TIME: 5 MINUTES, PLUS 5 HOURS TO MARINATE / COOK TIME: 25 MINUTES

This savory marinade that pairs gingery heat with garlicky goodness is simple, easy, and flavorful. It's a protein-rich juicy roast that is easy to scale up, so think of it as a spot-on party pleaser that pairs great with your favorite steamed or roasted veggies.

½ cup soy sauce (gluten-free, if desired) or liquid aminos

2 tablespoons Worcestershire sauce (gluten-free, if desired)

4 garlic cloves

4 tablespoons fresh ginger, chopped

1 (3-pound) pork tenderloin

1 In a blender or food processor, blend the soy sauce, Worcestershire sauce, garlic, and ginger until smooth.

2 Place the pork in a dish not much larger than the roast itself. Pour the marinade over the pork, cover, and marinate in the refrigerator for 4 hours. Remove the roast from the refrigerator 1 hour prior to roasting.

3 Preheat the oven to 425°F.

4 In a foil-lined baking dish, roast the pork for 20 to 25 minutes, until cooked through. Cooking time will vary based on thickness and diameter.

5 Remove from the oven and let rest for 10 minutes before carving and serving.

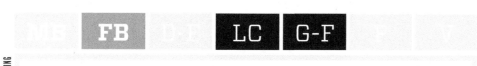

FB   LC   G-F

PER SERVING

Calories **110** Carbohydrates **0g** Fat **3g** Protein **22g**

4 ounces

PAN-SEARED SPICY GARLIC-GINGER PORK TENDERLOIN

MAKES 6 (4-OUNCE) SERVINGS / PREP TIME: 5 MINUTES /
COOK TIME: 30 MINUTES / TOTAL TIME: 45 MINUTES

Ideal for batch cooking

As soon as this tenderloin hits the pan, the aromas will surely make your mouth water. Searing activates the spices and seals in the moisture. Using a rub is a great way to add flavor without increasing calories.

FOR THE RUB

2 tablespoons garlic powder

2 tablespoons ground ginger

2 teaspoons ground cayenne pepper

1 teaspoon ground cumin

1 teaspoon salt

FOR THE PORK

1 (1½-pound) pork tenderloin, trimmed of excess fat

1½ teaspoons coconut oil

1 teaspoon minced garlic

1 tablespoon honey

Preheat the oven to 425°F.

TO MAKE THE RUB

In a small bowl, mix the garlic powder, ginger, cayenne, cumin, and salt.

TO PREPARE THE PORK

1 On a large plate, roll the tenderloin in the rub to coat.

2 In a large ovenproof skillet over medium-high heat, heat the coconut oil. Add the minced garlic, and cook, stirring, for 1 minute. Add the tenderloin, and cook, turning a few times, until lightly seared all around, about 5 minutes.

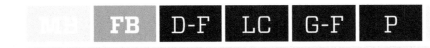

FB **D-F** **LC** **G-F** **P**

PER SERVING

Calories **128** Carbohydrates **3.8g** Fat **3.1g** Protein **24g**

4 ounces

3 Transfer the skillet to the oven, and roast for 20 to 25 minutes, turning over once halfway through cooking time, until cooked through. Cooking time will vary depending on the thickness of the meat.

4 Immediately drizzle the honey over the entire length of the tenderloin, and let rest for 5 to 10 minutes.

5 Using a sharp knife, slice the tenderloin against the grain into six equal pieces. Serve warm.

Time-saving tip: *To save prep time, the dry rub can be made in bulk and stored in a covered container at room temperature, ready for use the next time you make the dish.*

Cooking tip: *For a milder version, cut back on the cayenne.*

ALMOND-CRUSTED PORK CUTLETS

**MAKES 2 (4-OUNCE) SERVINGS / PREP TIME: 5 MINUTES /
COOK TIME: 10 MINUTES / TOTAL TIME: 20 MINUTES**

Comfort food made healthy, these cutlets are dredged in nutrient-dense ground almonds, instead of flour or breadcrumbs. Rather than deep-frying them, they're crisped up in a small amount of olive oil. Try adding Chunky Applesauce (page 205).

1 egg, lightly beaten

¼ cup almond flour

1 teaspoon Italian seasoning or dried oregano

Pinch salt

Pinch freshly ground black pepper

2 (4-ounce) boneless pork loin chops, trimmed of excess fat

1 tablespoon extra-virgin olive oil

Ingredient tip: If you don't have almond flour on hand, you can finely grind a handful of whole almonds in a food processor and blend into a flour.

1 In a shallow bowl, lightly beat the egg.

2 In a separate shallow bowl, mix the almond flour with the Italian seasoning, salt, and pepper.

3 Coat the pork chops in the egg, and then dredge the egg-coated pork in the almond flour mixture. Shake to remove any excess.

4 In a medium skillet over medium-high heat, heat the olive oil. Add the pork chops and cook, turning once, until golden brown and cooked through, about 5 minutes per side.

5 Transfer to plates and let rest for 5 minutes before serving.

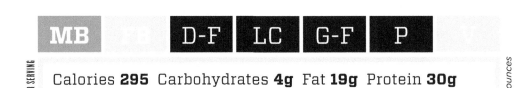

MB		D-F	LC	G-F	P

PER SERVING

Calories **295** Carbohydrates **4g** Fat **19g** Protein **30g**

4 ounces

HAM AND BEAN SOUP

**MAKES 10 (1½ CUP SERVINGS) / PREP TIME: 5 MINUTES /
COOK TIME: 25 MINUTES**

Ideal for batch cooking • Ideal for pre-workout

A bowl of this soup is a tasty dish with enough protein and slow-digesting carbs to fuel you through any workout. It can also be ready in minutes, a valuable bonus.

1 tablespoon extra-virgin olive oil

2 medium carrots, chopped

2 celery stalks, chopped

1 medium (about 4 ounces) white onion, chopped

4 (15-ounce) or 2 (28-ounce) cans cooked fava beans, drained and rinsed (7 cups)

4 cups low-sodium chicken broth

1½ pounds thickly sliced boneless ham, cut into cubes

1 teaspoon chili powder

1 dried bay leaf

½ teaspoon minced garlic

¼ teaspoon freshly ground black pepper

1 In a large, deep soup pot over medium-high heat, heat the olive oil.

2 Add the carrots, celery, and onion, and cook covered, stirring occasionally, until tender, about 10 minutes.

3 Add the beans, chicken broth, ham, chili powder, bay leaf, garlic, and pepper, and bring to a boil.

4 Turn the heat down to low, and simmer for 15 minutes.

5 Discard the bay leaf, ladle into soup bowls, and serve hot.

Time-saving tip: *This soup freezes well. Pack individual servings in airtight, freezer-safe containers and save for later.*

Ingredient tip: *You can substitute white beans for the fava beans. Keep in mind it will change the nutritional values.*

| MB | D-F | G-F | P |

PER SERVING

Calories **236** Carbohydrates **22.3g** Fat **5.1g** Protein **22.6g**

1½ cups

PORK AND MIXED-VEGETABLE STIR-FRY

MAKES 4 (4-OUNCE) SERVINGS / PREP TIME: 10 MINUTES / COOK TIME: 15 MINUTES

Chock-full of fiber, your gut and colon will thank you. A quick turn in the kitchen, this dish is great for a weeknight meal, or after a hard workout.

1 (1-pound) pork tenderloin, trimmed of excess fat

½ teaspoon ground ginger

¼ cup water

1 tablespoon granulated stevia

1 tablespoon cornstarch

12 ounces baby bok choy, root ends trimmed, stems and leaves chopped

2 medium carrots, chopped

1 red bell pepper, seeded and chopped

1 green bell pepper, seeded and chopped

2 tablespoons soy sauce (gluten-free if desired) or liquid aminos

1 teaspoon lemon zest plus 1 tablespoon freshly squeezed lemon juice

1 On a work surface, pat the tenderloin dry with paper towels. Using a sharp knife, slice the tenderloin against the grain into ½-inch-thick slices, and cut the slices into ½-inch strips.

2 Heat a large nonstick skillet over medium-high heat. If needed, coat very lightly with olive oil. Add the pork and ginger, and cook, stirring occasionally, for 5 minutes.

3 In a small bowl, mix the water with the stevia and cornstarch until the cornstarch has dissolved. Add the slurry to the pork, and stir to coat.

4 Add the baby bok choy, carrots, and red and green bell peppers to the skillet. Cover and cook for about 5 minutes, until the vegetables begin to soften.

5 Add the soy sauce, lemon zest, and lemon juice to the skillet. Cook, uncovered, stirring frequently, for 2 to 5 minutes more, until all of the vegetables are tender.

6 Divide the pork and vegetables among four plates, and serve.

FB D-F G-F

PER SERVING

Calories **181** Carbohydrates **12.8g** Fat **2.8g** Protein **25.8g**

4 ounces

PORK CHILE VERDE

**MAKES 6 (1-CUP) SERVINGS / PREP TIME: 15 MINUTES /
COOK TIME: 6 HOURS**

Hot peppers aren't just delicious, they're full of metabolism-boosting capsaicin that helps you feel full and burn more fat. You'll absolutely love how they heat things up.

1 (1½-pound) pork tenderloin, trimmed of excess fat and cut into 1-inch cubes

2½ cups low-sodium vegetable broth

1 bunch fresh cilantro, chopped

12 ounces Anaheim chiles, seeded and finely chopped

2 jalapeño peppers, seeded and finely chopped

1 large yellow onion (about 6 ounces), chopped

2 tablespoons minced garlic

2 teaspoons salt

1 teaspoon ground cumin

½ teaspoon freshly ground black pepper

½ teaspoon dried oregano

Pinch ground cloves

Lime wedges, for serving

1 In a slow cooker or a rice cooker with a slow cook setting, stir well to mix the pork, broth, cilantro, Anaheim chiles, jalapeños, onion, garlic, salt, cumin, black pepper, oregano, and cloves.

2 Cook on high for 6 hours.

3 Ladle into bowls and serve hot, with the lime wedges alongside. If you like, serve with a dollop of yogurt and a few cubes of chopped avocado (remember to add the calories to the total).

Time-saving tip: Depending on the size of your slow cooker, you can multiply the ingredients and feed a crowd. The dish also freezes well for future use.

FB	D-F	LC	G-F	P

PER SERVING

Calories **163** Carbohydrates **7.5g** Fat **2.5g** Protein **24.5g**

1 cup

HAWAIIAN-STYLE PORK AND PINEAPPLE SKEWERS

MAKES 10 SKEWERS / PREP TIME: 15 MINUTES, PLUS 15 MINUTES TO MARINATE / COOK TIME: 10 MINUTES

Ideal for post-workout • Ideal for batch cooking

Protein-full and sweet, tangy pineapple served up on a Hawaiian-style skewer, the simple sugars and powerful antioxidants in pineapple will help you recover from a tough training session. Enjoy these skewers with some rice for a high-carb post-workout meal, or with some steamed green veggies for a lighter option.

1 (2½-pound) pork tenderloin, trimmed of excess fat

2 (15-ounce) cans pineapple chunks in juice, drained, ½ cup of the juice reserved

½ cup apple cider vinegar

1½ teaspoons garlic powder

1 teaspoon ground ginger

½ teaspoon ground cayenne pepper

3 bell peppers, seeded and cut into 1-inch pieces

1 medium (about 4 ounces) red onion, cut into 1-inch pieces

1 pint cherry tomatoes

1 On a work surface, pat the tenderloin dry with paper towels. Using a sharp knife, cut the tenderloin against the grain into 1-inch-thick slices, and cut the slices into 1-inch cubes.

2 Tenderize the pork by piercing each cube with a fork in a few places.

3 In a small bowl, mix the reserved pineapple juice and vinegar with the garlic powder, ginger, and cayenne.

MB   **D-F**   **G-F**   **P**

PER SERVING

Calories **179** Carbohydrates **13g** Fat **2.7g** Protein **24.4g**

1 skewer

4 Put the cubed pork in a large resealable bag, add the marinade, seal the bag, and massage to coat the pork evenly. Marinate in the refrigerator for 15 minutes.

5 Thread the pork, pineapple chunks, bell peppers, onion, and tomatoes onto 10 skewers, alternating among the vegetables. For the sake of portions, spread the pork and pineapple evenly among the skewers, so that each skewer holds about 4 ounces of pork and 2 ounces of pineapple.

6 Preheat a grill to medium. Alternatively, preheat the oven broiler to high heat, set the rack about 8 inches from the heat, and line a broiler pan with aluminum foil.

7 Grill or broil the skewers, turning a few times, until the pork is lightly charred and cooked through, 8 to 12 minutes.

8 Serve warm.

FENNEL-CRUSTED ROAST PORK TENDERLOIN

MAKES 6 (4-OUNCE) SERVINGS / PREP TIME: 5 MINUTES / COOK TIME: 25 MINUTES / TOTAL TIME: 40 MINUTES

Ideal for batch cooking

Do you love breakfast sausage but avoid it because of its high calories? Here's a little gift: this calorie-free rub puts all the seasoning of a sausage on a lean, delicious tenderloin. Enjoy.

1½ teaspoons whole or ground fennel seeds

1½ teaspoons ground sage

1½ teaspoons garlic powder

1½ teaspoons onion powder

1½ teaspoons freshly ground black pepper

1 teaspoon dried parsley

½ teaspoon salt

1 (1½-pound) pork tenderloin, trimmed of excess fat

Time-saving tip: The dry rub keeps indefinitely in a covered container at room temperature. Make it in bulk and store for future use.

1 Preheat the oven to 425°F.

2 In a small bowl, mix the fennel seeds, sage, garlic powder, onion powder, pepper, parsley, and salt together to make a rub.

3 Line a rimmed baking sheet with aluminum foil or a silicone baking mat.

4 Pat the tenderloin dry with paper towels. Sprinkle the tenderloin with the rub, and massage well to coat. Set the tenderloin on the prepared baking sheet.

5 Bake for 20 to 25 minutes, turning once halfway through, until cooked through.

6 Transfer the pork to a cutting board and let rest for 10 minutes.

7 Using a sharp knife, slice the tenderloin against the grain into six equal portions.

8 Serve warm.

FB	D-F	LC	G-F	P

PER SERVING

Calories **120** Carbohydrates **0g** Fat **2.5g** Protein **23g**

4 ounces

COFFEE-RUBBED ROAST PORK TENDERLOIN

**MAKES 6 (4-OUNCE) SERVINGS / PREP TIME: 5 MINUTES /
COOK TIME: 25 MINUTES / TOTAL TIME: 40 MINUTES**

Ideal for pre-workout

Pork with a pick-me-up! This fat-burning rub of coffee and cayenne pepper boosts your energy levels, while adding a deep and rich flavor to the tenderloin—not to mention a kick from the hot pepper.

2 tablespoons ground coffee

1½ teaspoons ground cayenne pepper

1½ teaspoons salt

1 (1½-pound) pork tenderloin, trimmed of excess fat

¼ cup balsamic vinegar

1 Preheat the oven to 425°F.

2 In a small bowl, mix the coffee, cayenne, and salt together to make a rub.

3 Line a rimmed baking sheet with aluminum foil or a silicone baking mat.

4 Pat the tenderloin dry with paper towels. Sprinkle the tenderloin with the rub, and massage well to coat. Place the tenderloin on the prepared baking sheet.

5 Roast for 20 to 25 minutes, turning once halfway through, until cooked through.

6 Transfer to a cutting board and let rest for 10 minutes.

7 Using a sharp knife, slice the tenderloin against the grain into six equal portions, and transfer to a platter.

8 Drizzle the balsamic vinegar over the length of the sliced tenderloin, and serve immediately.

Time-saving tip: *If your tenderloin is rather thick, increase the roasting time by a few minutes.*

| FB | D-F | LC | G-F | P |

PER SERVING

Calories **129** Carbohydrates **1.8g** Fat **2.5g** Protein **23g**

4 ounces

CHAPTER SEVEN

FISH & SEAFOOD

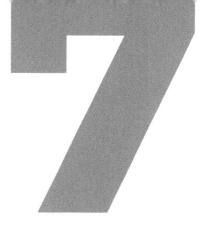

Whether you choose budget-friendly canned fish and crustaceans, or premier cuts from the counter, eating seafood not only seriously benefits your body, but is delicious, healthy, and ever so easy to prepare. White fish like cod, tilapia, ono, and mahimahi have juicy, firm flesh and are a great source of lean protein because they are very low in fat. Fatty fish like salmon and tuna are high in essential fatty acids and fat-soluble nutrients, like vitamin D, which are essential for your body, brain, and hormones to function optimally. A popular choice, shellfish, like shrimp, crab, and lobster, are a fantastically lean protein, rich in flavor and packed with valuable nutrients like zinc.

MB Muscle Building **FB** Fat Burning **D-F** Dairy-Free **LC** Low Carb **G-F** Gluten-Free **P** Paleo **V** Vegan

GARLIC AND HERB SHRIMP

MAKES 4 (4-OUNCE) SERVINGS /
PREP TIME: 5 MINUTES, PLUS 2 HOURS TO MARINATE / COOK TIME: 10 MINUTES
Ideal for batch cooking

A quick and easy way to enjoy succulent shrimp, loaded with lean protein. They turn out just the slightest bit sweet, and are packed with a ton of flavors.

1 pound medium-size shrimp, peeled, deveined, and tails on

1 tablespoon extra-virgin olive oil

1 tablespoon freshly squeezed lime juice

4½ teaspoons minced garlic

1 tablespoon granulated stevia

1 teaspoon ground paprika

1 teaspoon Italian seasoning

1 teaspoon dried basil

1 Put the shrimp, olive oil, lime juice, garlic, stevia, paprika, Italian seasoning, and basil in a large resealable bag. Massage the bag to ensure the shrimp are well coated. Marinate in the refrigerator for 2 hours.

2 Thread the shrimp onto skewers. If you are not using a rack, be sure to lightly spray the surface they are cooking on to prevent them from sticking.

3 To grill: Allow the barbecue to warm up to medium heat before placing the shrimp on the grill.

4 To broil: Set the oven rack about 8 inches from the broiler, line a broiler pan with aluminum foil, and arrange the shrimp skewers on it. Set your broiler to high and allow the oven to heat up a bit before placing the shrimp in it.

5 Cook the shrimp for 8 to 10 minutes, turning over once after 4 to 5 minutes. They are done when opaque with pink tails.

6 Serve warm.

Time-saving tip: Make your skewers based on your desired serving size. For 4-ounce servings, use 4 skewers per pound of shrimp, and so on.

FB D-F LC G-F P

PER SERVING

Calories **130** Carbohydrates **4g** Fat **3.9g** Protein **20g**
(4 ounces, about 9 medium shrimp)

SHRIMP CREOLE

MAKES 4 (4-OUNCE) SERVINGS / PREP TIME: 10 / COOK TIME: 1 HOUR

Ideal for pre-workout • Ideal for post-workout

Traditionally of Creole origin, this is guaranteed to become a family favorite. Serve it over rice for a great pre- or post-workout meal, or over steamed veggies for a leaner option.

1 tablespoon extra-virgin olive oil

½ cup (1 stalk) celery, chopped

½ cup (about 1 medium) onion, chopped

½ teaspoon minced garlic

1 (16-ounce) can petite diced tomatoes

1 (8-ounce) can tomato sauce

1 teaspoon soy sauce (gluten-free, if desired) or liquid aminos

1 teaspoon apple cider vinegar

¼ teaspoon freshly squeezed lemon juice

1½ teaspoons granulated stevia or honey

1½ teaspoons salt

½ teaspoon chili powder

2 teaspoons cornstarch

2 teaspoons water

½ cup (1 medium) green bell pepper, diced

1 pound jumbo shrimp, peeled and deveined

1 In a large skillet over medium-high heat, heat the olive oil. Add the celery, onion, and garlic, and cook until tender, but not brown, about 5 minutes.

2 Add the tomatoes, tomato sauce, soy sauce, apple cider vinegar, lemon juice, stevia, salt, and chili powder. Simmer uncovered for at least 20 minutes, and up to 45 minutes, stirring occasionally.

3 In a small bowl, mix the cornstarch and water. Stir the mixture into the skillet, and cook until the sauce is thick and bubbly.

4 Add the bell pepper and shrimp, cover, and simmer for 5 minutes more.

5 Divide among four bowls and enjoy.

Serving tip: *Shrimp Creole is best served over some rice. Try some chopped green onion and hot sauce for garnish. Remember to add the calories to the nutritional breakdown.*

MB   **D-F**   **G-F**

PER SERVING

Calories **168** Carbohydrates **11.8g** Fat **3g** Protein **22.3g**

4 ounces

COCONUT SHRIMP
WITH SWEET AND SPICY DIPPING SAUCE

**MAKES 6 SERVINGS / PREP TIME: 20 MINUTES /
COOK TIME: 15 MINUTES**

This one is a serious hit, because . . . coconut! And shrimp! Lean protein, coated in fiber and healthy fats from super-nutritious coconut flakes, makes this great as an appetizer, party snack, or a main dish.

FOR THE SHRIMP

3 tablespoons cornstarch

3 egg whites

6 tablespoons shredded coconut, unsweetened

2 tablespoons granulated stevia

24 medium shrimp, peeled, deveined, and tails on

FOR THE DIPPING SAUCE

¼ cup sugar-free orange marmalade

1 teaspoon sriracha

TO MAKE THE SHRIMP

1 Preheat the oven to 375°F.

2 Line a baking sheet with parchment paper.

3 Put the cornstarch in a small bowl.

4 In a second small bowl, whip the egg whites until stiff peaks form.

5 In a third small bowl, mix the coconut and stevia.

MB **D-F** **LC** **G-F**

PER SERVING

Calories **168** Carbohydrates **8.7g** Fat **3.5g** Protein **22.2g**

4 shrimp

6 Set the three bowls in a row. Take one shrimp by the tail, coat it in cornstarch, and then dip it in the whipped egg whites, the more volume the better. Finally, coat the shrimp in the coconut, and place it on the baking sheet.

7 Bake at 375°F for 10 to 15 minutes, turning over after about 7 minutes. The shrimp are done when the coconut has toasted and the tails are pink. (The egg white, if exposed, will still be white.)

TO MAKE THE DIPPING SAUCE

1 While the shrimp are in the oven, in a small bowl, mix the marmalade with the sriracha. If necessary, add a little water, 1 teaspoon at a time, to thin out the dipping sauce as needed.

2 Serve the shrimp warm with the dipping sauce.

HONEY-GARLIC SHRIMP

**MAKES 4 (4-OUNCE) SERVINGS /
PREP TIME: 5 MINUTES, PLUS 15 MINUTES TO MARINATE / COOK TIME: 2 MINUTES**

Ideal for post-workout

A touch of honey and garlic. A hint of ginger. Simple as it sounds, this sweet and savory shrimp dish shows that you don't need tons of ingredients to make a filling and delicious meal. This is great for refueling after a good workout.

¼ cup honey

2 tablespoons soy sauce (gluten-free, if desired) or liquid aminos

1 teaspoon garlic, minced

½ teaspoon ground ginger, minced

1 pound shrimp, peeled, deveined, and tails on

1 tablespoon coconut oil

1 In a large bowl, mix together the honey, soy sauce, garlic, and ginger. Transfer half of the mixture to another small bowl, and set aside.

2 Add the shrimp to the sauce in the large bowl, and toss to coat well. Marinate in the refrigerator for 15 minutes.

3 In a large skillet over medium-high heat, heat the coconut oil. Drain and discard any excess marinade from the shrimp, add the shrimp to the hot oil, and sear on both sides, about 1 minute per side, until the shrimp have slightly browned and the tails are pink. Remove from the heat.

4 Using a fork or tongs, rub the shrimp against the bottom of the skillet to collect the caramelized honey on the bottom of the pan.

5 Transfer to a plate, and drizzle with the remaining sauce. Divide among four plates and serve.

MB   **D-F**   **G-F**   **P**

PER SERVING

Calories **193** Carbohydrates **17.3g** Fat **4.5g** Protein **20g**

4 ounces

SHRIMP CEVICHE

MAKES 12 (4-OUNCE) SERVINGS /
PREP TIME: 20 MINUTES, PLUS 4 HOURS TO MARINATE / COOK TIME: 1 MINUTE
Ideal for batch cooking

Succulent shrimp in a spicy sea of fat-burning citrus, ceviche makes a great standalone snack or can be used instead of salsa on just about anything.

3 pounds shrimp, peeled and deveined

1 cup (from about 8½) freshly squeezed lime juice

1 cup (from 8 medium) freshly squeezed lemon juice

⅓ cup (from 1 medium) freshly squeezed orange juice

¼ cup (from ½ medium) freshly squeezed grapefruit juice

2 large tomatoes, diced

1 large red onion, diced

1 bunch fresh cilantro, chopped

1 jalapeño pepper, diced

2 large cucumbers, peeled and diced

2 large avocados, peeled, seeded, and diced

Ingredient tip: If you like your ceviche HOT, add a second jalapeño or 1 tablespoon ground cayenne pepper.

1 Place a large pot of water over high heat. Bring to a boil.

2 Put the shrimp in the boiling water for 45 seconds. Quickly pour the contents of the pot over a strainer in the sink, and then immediately transfer the shrimp to ice-cold water; this stops the cooking. Drain when cooled.

3 Chop the shrimp into ½-inch pieces and put them in a large bowl.

4 Pour the lime juice, lemon juice, orange juice, and grapefruit juice over the shrimp, and toss to coat.

5 Add the tomatoes, red onion, cilantro, and jalapeño, and toss gently. Cover and marinate in the refrigerator for 4 hours.

6 Add the cucumbers and avocados before serving.

FB **D-F** **G-F** **P**

PER SERVING

Calories **151** Carbohydrates **10.8g** Fat **3g** Protein **21g**

4 ounces

CIOPPINO

MAKES 8 (2-CUP) SERVINGS / PREP TIME: 30 MINS / COOK TIME: 50 MINS

Ideal for batch cooking

Cioppino, a fish stew from the San Francisco Bay Area, is one big tasty pot of protein. You can sub in fresh ingredients per your pantry: No fennel? Add three stalks of celery, or bok choy plus a dash of fennel seed for added flavor. Replace mahimahi with any other firm-fleshed white fish, like ono or halibut. You can also get creative and toss in some crab, calamari, or scallops.

1 tablespoon extra-virgin olive oil

1 large fennel bulb, thinly sliced

1 large white onion, chopped

3 large shallots, chopped

1 teaspoon salt (optional), plus more if desired

2 teaspoons minced garlic

1 teaspoon red pepper flakes, plus more if desired

¼ cup tomato paste

1 (28-ounce) can diced tomatoes in juice

5 cups fish stock

¾ cup freshly squeezed lemon juice

¾ cup water

1 dried bay leaf

1 pound Manila clams, scrubbed

1 pound mussels, scrubbed and debearded

1 pound large shrimp, peeled and deveined

1½ pounds mahimahi fillets, cut into 2-inch chunks

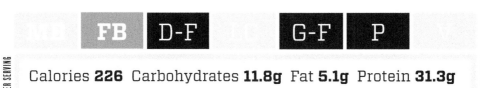

PER SERVING

FB D-F G-F P

Calories **226** Carbohydrates **11.8g** Fat **5.1g** Protein **31.3g**

≈ 2 cups

1 In a large soup pot over medium heat, heat the olive oil. Add the fennel, onion, shallots, and salt (if using), and cook for 10 minutes, stirring frequently, until the onion is translucent.

2 Add the garlic and red pepper flakes, and cook for 2 minutes more.

3 Stir in the tomato paste, tomatoes with their juices, fish stock, lemon juice, water, and bay leaf. Cover and bring to a simmer, and then reduce the heat to medium-low. Continue to simmer for 30 minutes.

4 Add the clams and mussels, cover, and cook for about 5 minutes, until the clams and mussels begin to open.

5 Add the shrimp and fish, and cook for about 5 minutes more, until the fish and shrimp are cooked through and the clams and mussels are completely open. Stir gently, careful not to break apart the fish.

6 Discard the bay leaf and any clams and mussels that failed to open.

7 Ladle a little of each shellfish, a little mahimahi, and some soup into each bowl, season with more salt and red pepper flakes as desired, and serve.

Ingredient tip: *When cleaning the clams and mussels, discard any that are already open.*

COCONUT-SEARED SCALLOPS
WITH WILTED SPINACH

SERVES 1 / PREP TIME: 5 MINUTES / COOK TIME: 10 MINUTES

Ideal for batch cooking

If you're looking for a first-class meal you can whip up in minutes, the mild, slightly sweet flavor of scallops provides a rich source of protein for a pleasing and nutritious main course. Seared in healthy coconut oil, with a serving of tender wilted baby spinach, this is a tasty meal you can feel good about.

FOR THE WILTED SPINACH
1½ teaspoons coconut oil
1 (10-ounce) bag baby spinach
Pinch freshly grated nutmeg

FOR THE SEARED SCALLOPS
1½ teaspoons coconut oil
4 jumbo sea scallops (about 4 ounces)
Salt

TO MAKE THE SPINACH

1 Heat a skillet over medium-high heat. Add the coconut oil, and swirl the skillet to coat the bottom.

2 Fill the skillet with spinach leaves. Cook, stirring, until wilted, about a minute. Add more spinach to the skillet, and repeat the process until all of the spinach is wilted.

3 Transfer the spinach to a plate, and lightly dust with nutmeg.

FB **D-F** **G-F** **P**

PER SERVING

Calories **277** Carbohydrates **12g** Fat **16g** Protein **25g**

TO MAKE THE SCALLOPS

1 Return the skillet to medium-high heat, add the coconut oil, and swirl to coat the bottom.

2 On a work surface, pat the scallops dry with paper towels, season with salt, and add to the skillet. Cook undisturbed for 1 to 2 minutes, until the bottoms brown. Flip, season with salt, and cook for another 1 to 2 minutes. They will be browned on both sides and cooked through but still slightly pink in the center.

3 Place the scallops atop the wilted spinach and enjoy.

Cooking tip: This meal cooks fast, so plan on making it fresh at the time you want to enjoy it. It is not a meal you want to reheat for leftovers. Feel free to get creative with some other spices. A light dusting of garlic powder or paprika or a squirt of lemon juice can really change the flavor.

Ingredient tip: It may seem like a lot of spinach, but once it all cooks down, it will only be about a cup of wilted spinach.

SCALLOP STIR-FRY

**MAKES 4 (4-OUNCE) SERVINGS / PREP TIME: 15 MINUTES /
COOK TIME: 10 MINUTES**

A member of the cruciferous family, bok choy is a delicious superfood high in carotenoids like beta-carotene and lutein. Pair it with these succulent scallops, and you'll have no problem fighting off free radicals. Enjoy by itself, or over rice.

FOR THE MARINADE

2 tablespoons soy sauce, (gluten-free, if desired) or liquid aminos

2 tablespoons freshly squeezed lemon juice

¼ cup rice vinegar

2 tablespoons honey

1 tablespoon cornstarch

2 teaspoons apple cider vinegar

1 garlic clove, crushed

Pinch freshly ground black pepper

FOR THE SCALLOPS

1 pound large scallops

1 teaspoon peanut oil or coconut oil

1 pound small baby bok choy, ends trimmed

1 pound white mushrooms, sliced

1 pound fresh snow peas

1 red bell pepper, cut into ½-inch pieces

1 onion, quartered, layers separated

MB   **D-F**   **G-F**

PER SERVING

Calories **171** Carbohydrates **22g** Fat **2.8g** Protein **15.8g**

4 ounces

TO MAKE THE MARINADE

In a small bowl, mix well to combine the soy sauce, lemon juice, rice vinegar, honey, cornstarch, apple cider vinegar, garlic, and pepper.

TO MAKE THE SCALLOPS

1 Pat the scallops dry with paper towels. In a medium bowl, drizzle the scallops with less than half of the marinade. Toss to coat.

2 Heat a large skillet over medium-high heat. Add the oil, and swirl to coat the pan. Add the scallops, and sear for 1 minute on each side. Remove and set aside.

3 Add the bok choy, mushrooms, snow peas, bell peppers, and onion to the skillet, and cook for about 5 minutes, until tender. Add the remaining marinade, and cook until heated through. Add the scallops back into the skillet, and cook for 1 more minute.

4 Divide among four plates and serve.

MAPLE AND MUSTARD–BAKED SCALLOPS

SERVES 1 / PREP TIME: 5 MINUTES / COOK TIME: 30 MINUTES

Ideal for batch cooking

Mouthwatering baked scallops with a sweet and tangy flavor, this great source of protein makes an excellent appetizer, snack, or protein topper for the Honey-Dijon Kale Salad (page 184).

4 jumbo sea scallops (about 4 ounces)
1½ teaspoons Dijon mustard
1½ teaspoons real maple syrup

Ingredient tip: *If you don't have maple syrup on hand, honey also works well— especially if you are serving them with the Honey-Dijon Kale Salad (page 184).*

Cooking tip: *Check the scallops often. No one likes an overcooked scallop.*

1 Preheat the oven to 350°F.

2 Place the scallops on a foil-lined baking sheet 1½ inches apart.

3 In a small bowl, mix the mustard and maple syrup. Spoon the mixture evenly over the scallops, and spread to coat the top.

4 Bake for 20 to 30 minutes, depending on size, until opaque.

5 Enjoy warm.

MB   **D-F**   **G-F**   **P**

PER SERVING

Calories **125** Carbohydrates **10g** Fat **1g** Protein **17g**

TUNA SALAD

SERVES 1 / PREP TIME: 5 MINUTES / COOK TIME: 5 MINUTES

Ideal for batch cooking

This tuna salad is so tasty you won't miss the mayo. Canned tuna is an affordable fish you don't have to fuss with. Nowhere else will you find 48 grams of protein at such a great price!

1 (7-ounce) can tuna in water, drained

1 tablespoon finely diced red onion

1 tablespoon finely diced dill pickle

1 tablespoon nonfat Greek yogurt

1½ teaspoons freshly squeezed lemon juice

1½ teaspoons extra-virgin olive oil

¼ teaspoon dried dill

Pinch freshly ground black pepper

2 tablespoons balsamic vinaigrette

1 In a small bowl, use a fork to mix the tuna, onion, pickle, yogurt, lemon juice, olive oil, dill, and pepper until well combined.

2 Drizzle the balsamic vinegar over the top and enjoy.

Ingredient tip: This recipe tastes even better as leftovers the next day.

Serving tip: Try enjoying it in a lettuce wrap or atop a bed of spinach.

FB　**LC**　**G-F**

PER SERVING

Calories **285** Carbohydrates **7g** Fat **8g** Protein **48g**

TUNA MELT–STUFFED TOMATOES

SERVES 2 / PREP TIME: 15 MINUTES / COOK TIME: 5 MINUTES

Super-high in protein and very low in cost, this breadless tuna melt with creamy Greek yogurt, a dash of mozzarella, and a hint of heat is the perfect filling lunch that won't leave you feeling weighed down.

1 (7-ounce) can tuna in water, drained

2 tablespoons nonfat Greek yogurt

1 tablespoon chopped fresh basil

1 tablespoon diced red bell pepper

1 tablespoon diced red onion

Pinch freshly ground black pepper

2 large tomatoes

¼ cup shredded low-fat mozzarella, divided

2 pinches crushed red pepper, divided

1 Preheat the broiler to high. In a small bowl, use a fork to mix the tuna, yogurt, basil, bell pepper, onion, and black pepper until well blended.

2 Slice off the top of each tomato with a sharp knife, and use a spoon to hollow out the tomatoes.

3 Stuff the tuna mixture into the tomato cups, and press down firmly with a fork.

4 Place the stuffed tomatoes in a loaf pan or baking dish. Top each with 2 tablespoons of shredded mozzarella and a pinch of crushed red pepper.

5 Broil 6 to 8 inches from the heat for 3 to 5 minutes, until the cheese melts and slightly browns.

6 Serve immediately. The stuffed tomatoes go well with salad greens or a veggie side dish.

FB   **G-F**

PER SERVING

Calories **189** Carbohydrates **10g** Fat **4g** Protein **31g**

1 stuffed tomato

ALMOND-CRUSTED BAKED COD

MAKES 4 (6-OUNCE) FILLETS / PREP TIME: 15 MINUTES / COOK TIME: 15 MINUTES

Decrease calories and preserve nutrition by baking, not frying, and using almond flour instead of wheat flour. Serve this cod up with homemade Sweet Potato Fries (page 208) for a healthy twist on fish and chips.

1 large egg

2 egg whites

½ cup blanched almond flour

½ teaspoon mustard powder

¼ teaspoon ground cayenne pepper

¼ teaspoon garlic powder

4 (6-ounce) cod fillets

Extra-virgin olive oil spray

1 Preheat the oven to 350°F.

2 Line a baking sheet with nonstick aluminum foil or a silicone baking mat.

3 In a medium bowl, whisk the egg and egg whites. Set aside.

4 In a large bowl, mix together the almond flour, mustard, cayenne pepper, and garlic powder.

5 On a work surface, pat the cod dry with paper towels. Dip a cod fillet into the egg, coating both sides. Shake off any excess. Dredge in the almond flour mixture, coating both sides, and place the seasoned cod on the prepared baking sheet. Repeat with the remaining cod.

6 Lightly spray each breaded fillet with olive oil spray. Bake for 15 minutes.

7 Plate the fish and serve fresh from the oven.

FB	D-F	LC	G-F	P

PER SERVING

Calories **245** Carbohydrates **3g** Fat **9.5g** Protein **36.5g**

1 6-ounce cod fillet

SALMON-QUINOA CAKES

MAKES 6 (3-CAKE) SERVINGS / PREP TIME: 15 MINUTES / COOK TIME: 30 MINUTES

Ideal for batch cooking • Ideal for pre-workout

The cheesiness in this good-for-you tasty little cake comes from nutritional yeast, deactivated yeast that looks like flakes and is available online, in the bulk food section of many grocery stores, or in some health food aisles. If you have leftover ingredients from your weekly meal prep, you can add them to the recipe, or replace with similar ingredients.

1 (7-ounce) can Alaskan salmon, undrained

1½ cups cooked quinoa

½ cup shredded (1 medium beet or 1½ medium carrots) raw beet or carrot

¼ cup finely diced onion, any color

1½ teaspoons minced garlic

½ teaspoon dried parsley or ¼ cup chopped fresh parsley

1 egg

2 egg whites

¼ cup nonfat Greek yogurt

¼ cup nutritional yeast

½ teaspoon salt

1 teaspoon coconut oil or extra-virgin olive oil

1 In a large bowl, stir together the salmon and its liquid with the quinoa. Add the beet, onion, garlic, and parsley, and mix well.

2 In a medium bowl, use a fork to beat the egg, egg whites, yogurt, nutritional yeast, and salt together.

3 Add the egg mixture to the salmon and quinoa mixture, and stir until well combined.

MB **G-F**

PER SERVING

Calories **160** Carbohydrates **14.5g** Fat **5.7g** Protein **13g**

3 cakes

4 Heat a large skillet over medium heat. Add the oil, and swirl to coat.

5 Using a ¼-cup measuring cup, scoop as many cakes into the skillet as will fit without the edges touching. Do not overcrowd. Fry for 5 to 8 minutes, until the bottoms brown and the cakes are firm. Flip and brown the other side, 3 to 5 minutes more.

6 Transfer to a dish to keep warm, and continue frying until all of the mixture has been used. The batter should make close to 18 cakes.

7 Serve warm.

Time-saving tip: *If you are in a rush to fry up the whole batch, have more than one skillet at a time going.*

GRILLED CALAMARI STEAKS
WITH MEDITERRANEAN TOPPING

SERVES 2 / PREP TIME: 15 MINUTES / COOK TIME: 5 MINUTES

Calamari steaks are a great lean protein option that cooks in a flash. You can make the salsa in bulk, then refrigerate in an airtight container for up to one week.

FOR THE TOPPING

¼ cup Kalamata olives, pitted and sliced

¼ cup Greek green olives, pitted and chopped

⅓ cup cherry tomatoes, chopped

2 tablespoons capers, drained

1½ teaspoons chopped fresh parsley

1½ teaspoons grated lemon zest, plus 1½ teaspoons freshly squeezed lemon juice

1 teaspoon minced garlic

Pinch freshly ground black pepper

FOR THE CALAMARI STEAKS

2 (6-ounce) calamari steaks

4½ teaspoons freshly squeezed lemon juice

1½ teaspoons extra-virgin olive oil

1½ teaspoons chopped fresh parsley

Salt

Freshly ground black pepper

Lemon wedges, for serving

FB	D-F	LC	G-F	P

PER SERVING

Calories **261** Carbohydrates **7g** Fat **15g** Protein **27.5g**

1 6-ounce steak

Preheat the grill to medium-high heat.

TO MAKE THE TOPPING

In a small bowl, stir together the olives, tomatoes, capers, parsley, lemon zest and juice, garlic, and pepper.

TO MAKE THE CALAMARI STEAKS

1 In a medium bowl, cover the calamari steaks with the lemon juice, olive oil, and parsley. Season with salt and pepper, and toss to combine.

2 Place the steaks directly over the heat on the grill. Grill the steaks for about 2 minutes on each side, until opaque. Do not overcook, or the calamari will be tough.

3 Top each calamari steak with half of the olive topping and a squeeze of lemon juice from the wedges, and serve.

Ingredient tip: *You can find calamari steak fresh or in the frozen food section. Defrost in the refrigerator overnight when you're ready to use them.*

"PARMESAN"-CRUSTED TILAPIA

**MAKES 2 (6-OUNCE) SERVINGS / PREP TIME: 5 MINUTES /
COOK TIME: 5 OR 15 MINUTES**

In this recipe, Parmesan is replaced with a healthier alternative: nutritional yeast. Not only does it have a delicious cheesy taste, it also provides 18 amino acids, including all nine essential ones, B-vitamins, iron, selenium, zinc, and fiber—a true nutritional powerhouse.

3 tablespoons nutritional yeast
1½ teaspoons extra-virgin olive oil
1½ teaspoons dried basil
¼ teaspoon salt
12 ounces tilapia fillets

In a small bowl, use a fork to stir the nutritional yeast, olive oil, dried basil, and salt into a paste. The paste will be grainy.

TO COOK IN THE OVEN

1 Preheat the oven to 350°F.

2 Place the fillets on a baking sheet lined with nonstick aluminum foil or on a silicone baking sheet. Spread the paste over the tops of each fillet, pressing it down into place.

3 Bake for 15 minutes, until the fish flakes easily when tested with a fork, and serve.

TO COOK IN THE MICROWAVE

1 Place the fillets on a microwave-safe dish. Spread the paste over the tops of each fillet, pressing it down into place.

2 Microwave on high for 4 to 5 minutes, depending on the size of the fillets, until the fish flakes easily when tested with a fork.

3 Allow them to rest for 1 to 2 minutes before serving.

Ingredient tip: Nutritional yeast is available online, in the bulk food section of many grocery stores, or in some health food aisles.

Serving tip: Try serving this over some undressed salad greens of kale, shredded Brussels sprouts, and shredded cabbage. The flavor of the fillets would complement a lot of dishes. Get creative!

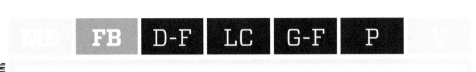

	FB	D-F	LC	G-F	P

PER SERVING

Calories **250** Carbohydrates **6g** Fat **8g** Protein **38g**

6 ounces

CRAB-STUFFED MUSHROOMS

MAKES 4 STUFFED MUSHROOMS / PREP TIME: 10 MINUTES / COOK TIME: 20 MINUTES

Between the sweet crab, nutty almond flour, cheesy nutritional yeast, and mushrooms you have a mouthful of nutrients in every bite. A serving is a great appetizer or snack; double or triple for a more filling meal.

2 tablespoons diced red onion

2 tablespoons diced celery

1 (6-ounce) can fancy crab meat, drained, or 4½ ounces fresh crab meat

2 tablespoons almond flour

2 tablespoons nutritional yeast

2 egg whites

¼ teaspoon mustard powder

Pinch ground paprika

Pinch ground cloves

4 medium (3-inch diameter) brown mushrooms, stems removed

¼ cup crisp rice cereal, crushed

Serving tips: Mushroom sizes can vary. For nutritional information, consider 1 serving to be half the total filling, the mushrooms it filled up, and 2 tablespoons of the crushed rice cereal.

If you are not a fan of mushrooms, try stuffing this mixture inside a bell pepper—or, for a fancier alternative, a broiled lobster tail!

1 Preheat the oven to 375°F.

2 In a small nonstick pan over medium-high heat, cook the onion and celery for about 5 minutes, until softened. Transfer to a small bowl.

3 Add the crab, almond flour, nutritional yeast, egg whites, mustard powder, paprika, and cloves to the bowl with the vegetables, and mix.

4 Place the mushroom caps on a baking sheet top down. Fill each with the crab mix, and sprinkle 1 tablespoon of the crushed rice cereal over the top.

5 Bake for 20 minutes, until the mushrooms are tender, and serve.

Ingredient tips: Nutritional yeast is available online, in the bulk food section of many grocery stores, or in some health food aisles.

If you don't have almond flour on hand, you can make some by grinding whole almonds into a flour.

| FB | D-F | LC | G-F | P |

PER SERVING

Calories **121** Carbohydrates **5g** Fat **3.5g** Protein **17.5g**

2 stuffed mushrooms

GRILLED ONO
WITH MANGO-PINEAPPLE SALSA

MAKES 2 SERVINGS / PREP TIME: 10 MINUTES, PLUS 20 MINUTE TO MARINATE / COOK TIME: 10 MINUTES

Hawaiian ono, also called wahoo, is a delicate, flaky, mild-flavored fish with a low fat content. It pairs perfectly with this tropical salsa made from some of the island's most delicious fruits.

FOR MARINATING THE ONO

4 (4-ounce) ono fillets

1 tablespoon coconut oil, melted

1 tablespoon freshly squeezed lime juice

¼ teaspoon garlic, minced

Dash ground cayenne pepper, plus more if desired

Dash salt

FOR THE SALSA

½ cup diced pineapple

½ cup (1 medium) peeled, pitted, and diced ripe mango

¼ cup diced red bell pepper

1 tablespoon minced red onion

1 tablespoon chopped fresh cilantro

1 tablespoon seeded and minced jalapeño pepper

Dash salt

Dash freshly ground black pepper

3 tablespoons freshly squeezed lime juice

FB **D-F** **LC** **G-F** **P**

PER SERVING

Calories **216** Carbohydrates **9g** Fat **6.3g** Protein **29.8g**

(4-ounce fillet with ⅔ cup salsa)

Preheat the grill to medium-high heat.

TO MARINATE THE ONO

1 Pat the ono dry with paper towels, and put in a large resealable bag.

2 In a small bowl, mix well to combine the coconut oil, lime juice, garlic, cayenne pepper, and salt. Pour into the resealable bag with the fish. Seal the bag, and gently massage to ensure the fillets are well coated. Marinate in the refrigerator for 20 minutes.

TO MAKE THE SALSA

In a small bowl, mix well to combine the pineapple, mango, bell pepper, onion, cilantro, jalapeño, salt, and pepper. Drizzle the lime juice over and toss.

TO GRILL THE FISH

1 Grill the ono for about 4 minutes on each side. The fish is done when it is opaque and flakes easily with a fork.

2 Serve each fillet topped with ⅔ cup of the salsa.

Time-saving tip: This salsa can be prepared in bulk to have on hand for other meals. Fresh fruit is best, but you can always opt for no-sugar-added canned fruit to save the time spent peeling and dicing.

BROILED SALMON
WITH INDIAN SPICES

**MAKES 4 (6-OUNCE) SERVINGS / PREP TIME: 5 MINUTES /
COOK TIME: 10 MINUTES**

Surprise your taste buds with something new! This spice blend really complements the salmon, and when broiled, it creates a perfect crust on the outside while keeping the fish tender and juicy on the inside. Try pairing it with some Cucumber Salad (page 178).

Extra-virgin olive oil spray
½ teaspoon ground coriander
½ teaspoon garam masala
½ teaspoon ground ginger
¼ teaspoon ground turmeric
Dash salt
Dash ground red pepper
4 (6-ounce) skinless salmon fillets

1 Preheat the broiler.

2 Line a baking sheet with nonstick aluminum foil, and lightly spray the foil with olive oil spray.

3 In a small bowl, mix the coriander, garam masala, ginger, turmeric, salt, and red pepper.

4 Place the fillets on the lined baking sheet, and rub the spice mixture evenly over each fillet.

5 Loosely cover with foil, and broil 4 to 6 inches from the flame for about 7 minutes.

6 Remove the foil and broil for about 3 minutes more, to desired degree of doneness.

FB | **D-F** | **LC** | **G-F** | **P**

PER SERVING

Calories **150** Carbohydrates **3g** Fat **1.5g** Protein **31.5g**

6 ounces

GRILLED BALSAMIC AND ROSEMARY SALMON

**MAKES 4 (4-OUNCE) SERVINGS /
PREP TIME: 5 MINUTES, PLUS 30 MINUTES TO MARINATE / COOK TIME: 10 MINUTES**

Quick to grill and delicious to eat, this healthy grilled salmon pairs great with Garlicky Roasted Brussels Sprouts (page 192) or Protein Mashed Potatoes (page 196).

4 (4-ounce) salmon fillets

Salt

3 tablespoons balsamic vinegar

2 tablespoons freshly squeezed
   lemon juice

1 tablespoon extra-virgin olive oil,
   plus more for oiling the grate

1 teaspoon minced garlic

2 tablespoons minced fresh
   rosemary, divided

1 In a small glass baking dish just big enough to hold the salmon fillets, sprinkle the fillets with salt.

2 In a small bowl, whisk together the vinegar, lemon juice, olive oil, and garlic. Pour the mixture over the salmon fillets.

3 Sprinkle 1 tablespoon of the minced rosemary over the top of the fillets, cover, and marinate in the refrigerator for at least 30 minutes.

4 Preheat the grill to medium-high heat, and lightly oil the grate.

5 Remove the salmon from the marinade, and discard any remaining marinade. Grill for 4 minutes on each side, until the fish is opaque in the center and flakes easily with a fork.

6 Transfer to a platter, sprinkle with the remaining tablespoon of minced rosemary, and serve.

FB	D-F	LC	G-F	P

PER SERVING

Calories **117** Carbohydrates **3g** Fat **2g** Protein **21g**

4 ounces

MAHIMAHI TACOS
WITH CILANTRO-LIME CREMA

MAKES 8 TACOS / PREP TIME: 15 MINUTES / COOK TIME: 10 MINUTES

Ideal for pre-workout

This taco is sure to become a favorite! Flaky pieces of white fish covered in a piquant rub and drizzled with creamy-tangy topping is a proposition hard to resist. The recipe makes enough to share, and offers a good balance of macronutrients to fuel your workout.

Extra-virgin olive oil spray

FOR THE CREMA
¼ cup thinly sliced green onions
¼ cup chopped fresh cilantro
¼ cup nonfat Greek yogurt
2 teaspoons extra-virgin olive oil
1 teaspoon grated lime zest, plus
    2 teaspoons freshly squeezed
    lime juice
¼ teaspoon salt
½ teaspoon minced garlic

FOR THE MAHIMAHI
1 teaspoon ground coriander
1 teaspoon ground cumin
½ teaspoon ground smoked paprika
¼ teaspoon ground red pepper
⅛ teaspoon salt
⅛ teaspoon garlic powder
4 (6-ounce) mahimahi fillets

FOR THE TACOS
8 (6-inch) corn tortillas
2 cups shredded cabbage
Lime wedges

MB　　**G-F**

PER SERVING

Calories **159**　Carbohydrates **10.8g**　Fat **4.9g**　Protein **17.8g**

(1 taco with 3 ounces of fish)

1 Preheat the oven to 425°F.

2 Line a baking sheet with nonstick aluminum foil, and lightly coat the foil with olive oil spray.

TO MAKE THE CREMA

In a small bowl, mix together the green onions, cilantro, yogurt, olive oil, lime zest and juice, salt, and garlic, and set aside.

TO MAKE THE MAHIMAHI

1 In a small bowl, mix together the coriander, cumin, paprika, red pepper, salt, and garlic powder.

2 Place the fillets on the prepared baking sheet. Sprinkle the spice mixture evenly over both sides of each mahi-mahi fillet, and pat it gently into place.

3 Bake for about 10 minutes, until opaque and flakes easily with a fork.

TO ASSEMBLE THE TACOS

1 Heat the tortillas according to package directions.

2 Place two corn tortillas on a plate, and divide one (6-ounce) fillet between them, gently breaking the fillet apart with a fork into large flakes. Top each taco with ¼ cup of cabbage and 1 tablespoon of crema. Garnish with lime wedges.

3 Repeat with the remaining ingredients and serve.

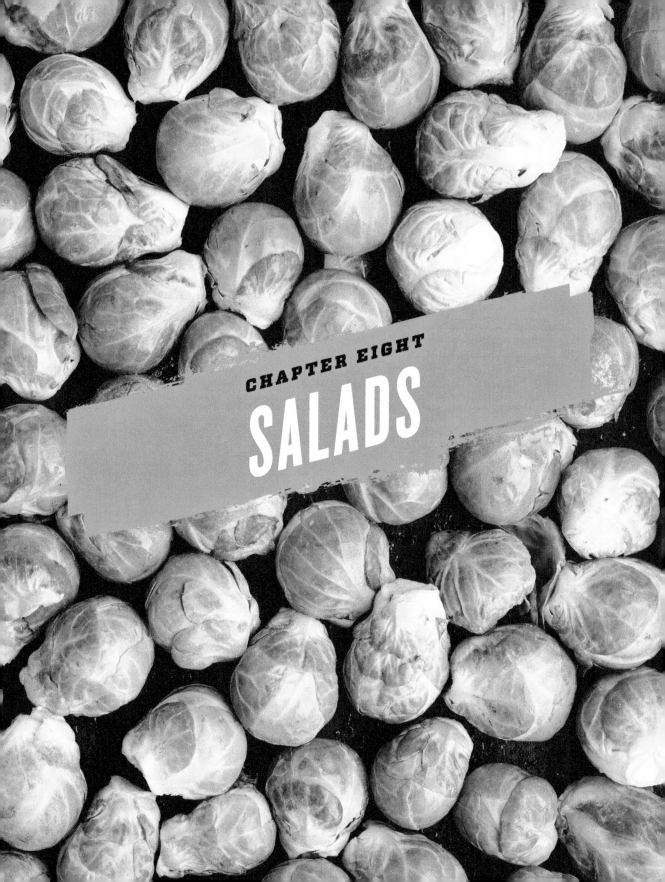

CHAPTER EIGHT

SALADS

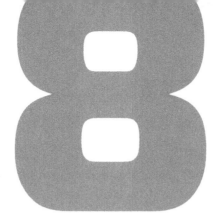

Ingredients that build muscle, burn fat, and are mouthwatering while not wasting calories ... what's not to love? If you are not inclined to eat your daily vegetables, making one of your meals a salad is a super-easy way to guarantee you get enough of them. In general, vegetables in salads are good sources of the insoluble fiber that keeps your belly full and your digestive tract healthy. Salads with a variety of veggies include all kinds of antioxidants, vitamins, minerals, and phytochemicals. The infinite ingredient combinations allow you to create a meal that has whatever macronutrient ratios and flavors your body is craving.

MB Muscle Building **FB** Fat Burning **D-F** Dairy-Free **LC** Low Carb **G-F** Gluten-Free **P** Paleo **V** Vegan

CUCUMBER SALAD

MAKES 5 SERVINGS / PREP TIME: 15 MINUTES

Ideal for batch cooking

Light and refreshing, with a sweet and tangy flavor that really hits the spot, this salad is unbelievably filling, considering how few calories are in each serving! Try it with the Spicy Turkey Satay Skewers (page 73).

2 seedless cucumbers

1 medium red onion

1 bunch fresh cilantro, chopped

½ cup granulated stevia

½ cup rice vinegar

2 tablespoons freshly squeezed lime juice

½ cup unsalted roasted cashews, whole or chopped, divided (optional)

Time-saving tip: *Divide the salad among five meal prep containers for a week's worth of salad.*

1 Slice the cucumber into thin rounds using a mandoline slicer, or knife.

2 Quarter the onion, and thinly slice with a mandoline slicer, or knife.

3 In a large bowl, toss the cucumber, onion, and cilantro.

4 In a small bowl, mix the stevia, vinegar, and lime juice until the stevia is dissolved.

5 Add the dressing to the salad, and toss to coat.

6 Divide the salad among five salad plates, garnish each with about 1½ tablespoons of cashews (if using), and serve.

FB	D-F	G-F	V

PER SERVING

Calories **28** Carbohydrates **6.7g** Fat **0g** Protein **1g**   =1 cup w/o nuts

Calories **103** Carbohydrates **10.6g** Fat **6g** Protein **3.2g**   =1 cup w nuts

CHICKEN WALDORF SALAD

SERVES 4 / PREP TIME: 5 MINUTES /
COOK TIME: 15 MINUTES / TOTAL TIME: 25 MINUTES

A well-balanced meal, this salad will keep you satisfied for hours. The lean protein from chicken breast is boosted by protein-rich Greek yogurt and vitamin powerhouses, walnuts and salad greens.

16 ounces boneless, skinless chicken breasts, cubed

2 cups celery stalks, chopped

1½ cups (3 medium) chopped Granny Smith apples

½ cup nonfat Greek yogurt

1 tablespoon freshly squeezed lemon juice

¼ cup Medjool dates, chopped

¼ cup walnuts, chopped

1 tablespoon salt

3 tablespoons granulated stevia

8 cups salad greens, divided

Cooking tip: If you have time, leave the finished chicken salad in the fridge for a few hours before topping the salad greens so the flavors can blend.

1 Preheat the oven to 350°F.

2 Place the chicken breasts on a nonstick pan, and bake for 10 to 15 minutes, until the chicken is cooked through. Cooking time will vary based on the size of the breasts.

3 Let the chicken cool, and cut into cubes.

4 In a large bowl, toss the chicken, celery, and apples. In a small bowl, mix the yogurt and lemon juice. Add the yogurt mixture to the chicken mixture, and toss to coat.

5 Add the dates and walnuts, and toss. Season with the salt and stevia.

6 Put about 2 cups of the mixed greens on each of 4 large serving plates, and top each with one-quarter of the chicken mixture. Serve cold and enjoy!

MB   **G-F**

PER SERVING

Calories **265** Carbohydrates **17.6g** Fat **9.2g** Protein **29.9g**   ≈1 cup

BRUSSELS SPROUTS AND BERRIES SALAD

SERVES 1 / PREP TIME: 20 MINUTES

Ideal for batch cooking • Ideal for pre-workout

Brussels sprouts aren't just super nutritious, they are durable. This is one salad that will not get soggy and will travel well. Berries can improve performance, so enjoy this salad before heading to the gym.

FOR THE DRESSING

1½ teaspoons extra-virgin olive oil
½ teaspoon honey
½ teaspoon apple cider vinegar
¼ teaspoon grated lemon zest, plus ¼ teaspoon freshly squeezed lemon juice
¼ teaspoon brown mustard
⅛ teaspoon garlic powder
Salt
Freshly ground black pepper

FOR THE SALAD

½ pound Brussels sprouts, shredded (approximately 3 cups)
1 tablespoon dried blueberries or ¼ cup fresh
1 tablespoon dried cranberries
1 tablespoon chopped almonds

TO MAKE THE DRESSING

In a small bowl, whisk well to combine the olive oil, honey, apple cider vinegar, lemon zest and juice, brown mustard, and garlic powder, and season with salt and pepper.

TO MAKE THE SALAD

1 In a large bowl, drizzle the dressing on top of the Brussels sprouts and toss well.

2 Add the blueberries, cranberries, and almonds, toss gently, and enjoy.

Ingredient tip: *Many stores carry Brussels sprouts already shredded. If you are working with whole Brussels sprouts, use a food processor or blender to shred them quickly.*

MB	D-F	G-F	P	V

PER SERVING

Calories **209** Carbohydrates **23g** Fat **12g** Protein **3g**

SALMON SALAD

SERVES 4 / PREP TIME: 10 MINUTES

Ideal for batch cooking

Not only does salmon give you a sizable serving of protein, the fatty acids also help your body and mind achieve optimal performance. Serve this deliciousness over a bed of salad greens to take advantage of their filling fiber and various nutrients.

3 (7-ounce) cans boneless, skinless salmon, drained

3 celery stalks, finely chopped

⅓ cup diced red onion

1 tablespoon dried dill

2 tablespoon capers or minced dill pickle

2 tablespoon apple cider vinegar

½ teaspoon salt (optional)

½ teaspoon freshly ground black pepper

1 In a large bowl, gently break the salmon into large flakes with a fork.

2 Add the celery, onion, dill, capers, vinegar, salt (if using), and pepper, and mix well.

3 Divide among four plates and serve, either alone or on a bed of your favorite salad greens.

Ingredient tip: If you prefer fresh salmon instead of canned, cook it ahead of time and allow it to cool completely in the refrigerator before preparing the salad.

MB **D-F** **LC** **G-F** **P**

PER SERVING

Calories **174** Carbohydrates **1.2g** Fat **7.5g** Protein **26.3g**

≈1 cup

CITRUS-BEET SALAD
WITH TOASTED WALNUTS

SERVES 6 / PREP TIME: 10 MINUTES

Ideal for pre-workout • Ideal for batch cooking

This salad is overflowing with flavor and nutrients to power your workout. Citrus and vinegar flavors balance the sweetness of the roasted beets, while tangerines temper the bite of the salad greens. Top with your favorite protein, like chicken or beef, for a complete meal.

FOR THE DRESSING

¼ cup orange juice

1 tablespoon apple cider vinegar

1 teaspoon granulated stevia

¼ teaspoon salt

¼ teaspoon freshly ground
   black pepper

½ teaspoon minced garlic

FOR THE SALAD

3 cups sliced baked beets
   (see page 207)

9 cups mixed salad greens, divided

6 tangerines, peeled and sectioned,
   divided

3 tablespoons toasted walnuts,
   coarsely chopped, divided

MB		D-F		G-F	P	V

PER SERVING

Calories **130** Carbohydrates **23g** Fat **3g** Protein **4g**

≈1 cup

TO MAKE THE DRESSING

In a small bowl, mix well to combine the orange juice, apple cider vinegar, stevia, salt, pepper, and garlic.

TO MAKE THE SALAD

1 In a medium bowl, pour the dressing over the beets and toss to coat evenly.

2 Put 1½ cups mixed salad greens on each plate, and top with ½ cup of the beets, the sections of 1 tangerine, and 1½ teaspoons of toasted walnuts.

3 Drizzle a little dressing from the bowl of beets over the top and serve.

Time-saving tip: To pack this salad up in meal prep containers, divide the beets into ½-cup portions, and distribute any remaining dressing evenly among the six containers. Package the 1½ cup salad greens and ½ tablespoon toasted walnuts in a separate container. When you are ready to enjoy the salad, combine the mixed greens with the beets. Peel the tangerine, and place the slices on top. Doing it this way will prevent the salad from getting soggy.

Ingredient tips: If you don't have any baked beets on hand, you can use 3 cups of canned beets instead. They are not as flavorful, but they still get the job done.

You can easily toast your own walnuts by baking them for 5 to 10 minutes in a 375°F oven.

HONEY-DIJON KALE SALAD

SERVES 4 / PREP TIME: 20 MINUTES

Ideal for post-workout

Cranberries, apples, and sweet honey mustard will help refuel your muscles after a tough workout. This salad is great topped with chicken.

FOR THE SALAD

8 ounces kale, stemmed and chopped

Pinch salt

1 medium Granny Smith apple, cored and chopped

4 medium radishes, thinly sliced

½ cup dried cranberries

½ cup toasted pecans, chopped

1 ounce soft goat cheese, crumbled

FOR THE DRESSING

1 tablespoon extra-virgin olive oil

1 tablespoon water

4½ teaspoons apple cider vinegar (or white wine vinegar)

1 tablespoon Dijon mustard

1½ teaspoons honey

Salt

Freshly ground black pepper

TO MAKE THE SALAD

1 In a large bowl, mix the kale and salt, massaging the leaves with your hands until the leaves are darker in color and fragrant, about 5 minutes.

2 Add the apple, radishes, cranberries, pecans, and goat cheese to the bowl.

TO MAKE THE DRESSING

1 In a small bowl, whisk together the olive oil, water, apple cider vinegar, mustard, and honey, and season with salt and pepper. Pour the dressing over the salad, and toss to coat.

2 Divide among four plates and serve.

Cooking tip: For better flavor, let the salad marinate in the dressing for 10 to 20 minutes before serving.

Ingredient tip: You can easily toast your own pecans by baking them in a 350°F oven for 5 to 10 minutes.

MB   **G-F**

PER SERVING

Calories **262** Carbohydrates **32.2g** Fat **15.2g** Protein **5.2g**

≈1 cup

SPINACH CAPRESE SALAD

SERVES 1 / PREP TIME: 5 MINUTES

This simple and satisfying salad makes a perfect side dish to any Italian entrée. Fibrous spinach will keep you full and satisfied. The combination of ingredients will give you a balanced meal with protein, healthy fats, vegetable-based carbohydrates, and a ton of vitamins and minerals. Make a single serving for yourself, or multiply the ingredients to feed an army of guests!

1½ cups baby spinach
½ cup cherry tomatoes, quartered
1 ounce fresh mozzarella, cubed
2 tablespoons chopped fresh basil
4½ teaspoons extra-virgin olive oil
1 tablespoon balsamic vinegar
Salt
Freshly ground black pepper

1 In a salad bowl, sprinkle the cherry tomatoes, mozzarella, and basil over the baby spinach.

2 Drizzle the olive oil and balsamic over the top, season with salt and pepper, and enjoy.

FB   **LC** **G-F**

PER SERVING

Calories **181** Carbohydrates **8g** Fat **12g** Protein **19g**

MEDITERRANEAN BEAN SALAD

MAKES 10 (1-CUP) SERVINGS / PREP TIME: 10 MINUTES, PLUS 1 HOUR TO CHILL

Ideal for batch cooking

With the fiber and slow-digesting carbohydrates in the various beans, this salad can stabilize your blood sugar for hours. Pair it with your favorite lean cut of meat and vegetable side dish for a balanced meal.

FOR THE VINAIGRETTE

3 tablespoons red wine vinegar

3 tablespoons extra-virgin olive oil

2 tablespoons water

1 teaspoon dried oregano

1 teaspoon minced garlic

1 teaspoon Dijon mustard

½ teaspoon salt

1 teaspoon freshly ground
    black pepper

FOR THE SALAD

1 (15.5-ounce) can cannellini beans,
    rinsed and drained

1 medium fennel bulb (approximately
    8 ounces), chopped

2 medium red onions (approximately
    8 ounces total), thinly sliced

1 cup canned pitted ripe olives,
    drained and halved

¾ cup chopped fresh parsley

2 cups cherry tomatoes, halved

½ cup feta cheese, crumbled

2 tablespoons sunflower seeds

½ cup pepperoncini, diced (optional)

TO MAKE THE VINAIGRETTE

In a small bowl, mix together the vinegar, olive oil, water, oregano, garlic, mustard, salt, and pepper.

TO MAKE THE SALAD

1 In a large bowl, toss to combine the beans, fennel, onions, olives, parsley, tomatoes, and feta. Pour the vinaigrette on top, and toss again.

2 Sprinkle the salad with the feta, sunflower seeds, and pepperoncini (if using). Cover and refrigerate for at least 1 hour to allow the flavors to meld.

3 Serve on its own, on a bed of mixed greens, or as a side dish.

MB   **G-F**

PER SERVING

Calories **141** Carbohydrates **18.4g** Fat **6.3g** Protein **6.1g**

1 cup

SOUTHWESTERN SALAD
WITH PULLED CHICKEN AND CILANTRO-LIME DRESSING

SERVES 1 / PREP TIME: 30 MINUTES

Ideal for pre-workout

This salad is a complete meal with all the macros you need—including a whopping 51 grams of protein!—in one delicious bowl. Your mouth will have a Southwestern fiesta when it encounters the delicate aromas of creamy cilantro dressing drizzled over succulent pulled chicken and lush avocado.

FOR THE DRESSING

1 cup fresh cilantro leaves

¼ cup nonfat Greek yogurt

½ teaspoon minced garlic

2 tablespoons freshly squeezed lime juice

1 tablespoon extra-virgin olive oil

1 tablespoon apple cider vinegar

FOR THE SALAD

3 cups chopped romaine lettuce

¼ cup canned black beans, drained and rinsed

6 ounces Pulled Chicken (page 72)

¼ cup cherry tomatoes, halved

¼ avocado, diced

2 tablespoons salsa

2 tablespoons fresh cilantro leaves, chopped

TO MAKE THE DRESSING

In a food processor or blender, process the cilantro leaves, yogurt, garlic, lime juice, olive oil, and apple cider vinegar until smooth. If too thick, add water in small increments and process to desired thickness. Refrigerate while preparing the salad.

TO MAKE THE SALAD

1 In a large bowl, evenly spread the black beans and Pulled Chicken on top of the romaine. Sprinkle the tomatoes and avocado over the salad.

2 Drizzle the dressing over the salad, garnish with the salsa and cilantro leaves, and enjoy.

MB

G-F

PER SERVING

Calories **477** Carbohydrates **26g** Fat **21g** Protein **51g**

THAI PEANUT SALAD

SERVES 1 / PREP TIME: 15 MINUTES

Irresistible peanut flavor without the calories that go with it, this Thai dressing is packed with lean protein. It might look like a lot of carbs, but they are all coming from healthy, fibrous veggies. Try this salad topped with chicken or shrimp.

FOR THE THAI PEANUT DRESSING
¼ cup defatted peanut flour
2 tablespoons rice vinegar
2 tablespoons freshly squeezed
   lime juice
1 tablespoon soy sauce (gluten-free,
   if desired) or liquid aminos
2 tablespoons honey
1 teaspoon minced garlic
¼ teaspoon ground ginger
½ teaspoon salt
¼ teaspoon crushed red pepper flakes

FOR THE SALAD
3 cups chopped napa cabbage or
   shredded coleslaw mix
1 cup shredded carrots
1 red bell pepper, cut into thin,
   bite-size pieces
2 medium green onions, thinly sliced
½ cup loosely packed chopped
   fresh cilantro

TO MAKE THE DRESSING
In a small bowl, mix together the flour, vinegar, lime juice, soy sauce, honey, garlic, ginger, salt, and red pepper flakes. Refrigerate until ready to serve.

TO MAKE THE SALAD
1 In a large bowl, toss together the cabbage, carrots, bell pepper, green onions, and cilantro.

2 Drizzle the dressing over the salad, toss again, and enjoy.

Time-saving tip: Prepare the dressing in bulk and store in the fridge. Stir before using.

Cooking tip: Packing your salad for later? Store the dressing separately so the salad doesn't get soggy.

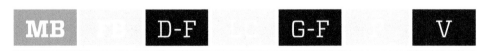

PER SERVING

Calories **246** Carbohydrates **50g** Fat **1g** Protein **16g**

CURRY QUINOA SALAD

SERVES 6 / PREP TIME: 10 MINUTES / COOK TIME: 15 MINUTES

Ideal for pre-workout • Ideal for batch cooking

This Indian-inspired salad with the protein- and fiber-rich quinoa makes a great side dish alternative to rice, and is even more amazing when topped with your favorite protein.

1 teaspoon extra-virgin olive oil

2 teaspoons curry powder or Madras curry powder

1 teaspoon minced garlic

1 cup quinoa

2 cups water

½ teaspoon salt

1 mango, peeled and diced

½ cup diced celery

¼ cup thinly sliced green onion

3 tablespoons chopped fresh cilantro

¼ cup finely diced cucumber

2 teaspoons chopped fresh mint

1 cup nonfat Greek yogurt

1 (5-ounce) package fresh baby spinach

Time-saving tip: *To pack this salad up in meal prep containers, divide the spinach evenly among 6 meal prep containers, and top each with about ¾ cup quinoa mixture and about 2 tablespoons yogurt mixture.*

1 In a medium saucepan over medium-high heat, heat the olive oil. Add the curry and garlic, and cook for 1 minute, stirring constantly.

2 Add the quinoa and water, and bring to a boil. Cover, reduce the heat, and simmer for 15 minutes, or until tender and no water remains.

3 Remove from heat, stir in the salt, and set aside to cool.

4 Once the quinoa has cooled completely, add the mango, celery, green onion, and cilantro. Toss gently.

5 In a small bowl, stir well to combine the cucumber, mint, and yogurt.

6 Put some spinach on each plate, top each with about ¾ cup quinoa mixture and 2 tablespoons yogurt mixture, and serve.

Ingredient tip: *Madras curry will make the dish spicier than regular curry powder.*

MB　　　**G-F**

PER SERVING

Calories **168** Carbohydrates **28.3g** Fat **2.6g** Protein **8.3g**

(¾ cup quinoa, 2 tablespoons yogurt mix, handful spinach)

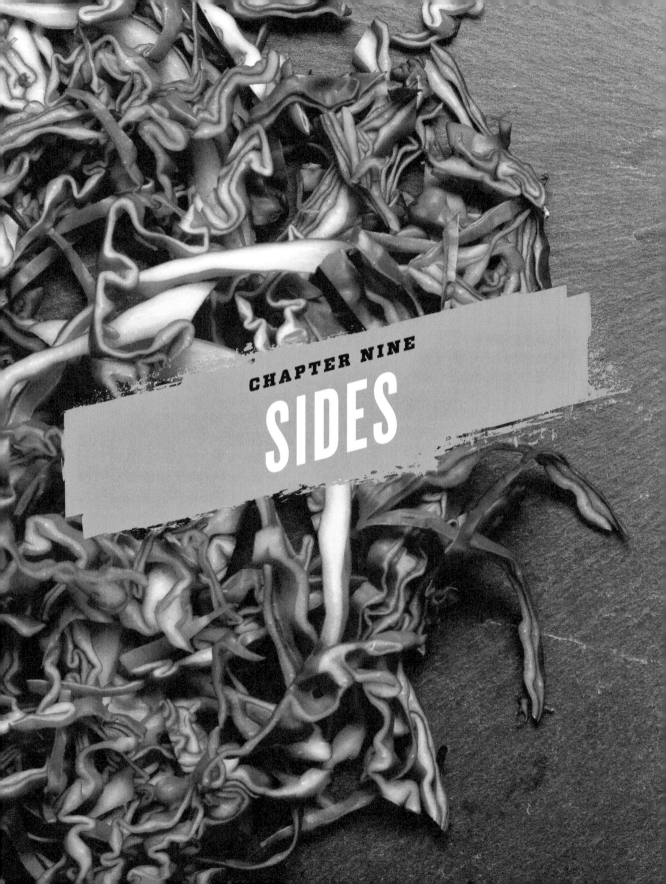

CHAPTER NINE

SIDES

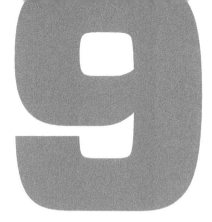

The bodybuilding diet is notorious for its boring side dishes. For too long, the fitness-minded have suffered, trying to choke down another bowlful of steamed broccoli and brown rice. Well, my friends, I am here to offer you salvation. In this chapter you will find 16 easy flavor-packed recipes to banish boring for good. By adding any of these side dishes to an ordinary piece of protein, you can transform a typical meal into a memorable one. Sweet, savory, salty, spicy, nutty, tangy, or tart; no matter what you are craving, there is a recipe here that will tantalize your taste buds. Vegetables and complex carbs provide an abundance of valuable nutrients that are essential to any fitness regimen. No supplement can hold a candle to their vitamins, minerals, and fiber—keys for growth and energy. But that doesn't mean we have to endure them like we do a workout. Whether you are making dinner for the family or preparing food for the week, add these excellent side dishes to the menu. Now you can finally look forward to eating your veggies!

MB Muscle Building **FB** Fat Burning **D-F** Dairy-Free **LC** Low Carb **G-F** Gluten-Free **P** Paleo **V** Vegan

GARLICKY ROASTED BRUSSELS SPROUTS

MAKES 5 CUPS / PREP TIME: 5 MINUTES / COOK TIME: 1 HOUR

Ideal for batch cooking

Packed with flavor, these super veggies deliver a hefty dose of vitamins, minerals, and phytonutrients for very few calories—and hardly any work. Eating just a few Brussels sprouts will give you a full dose of fiber, lots of vitamins, including A, C, and B-6, plus a good amount of minerals, such as potassium, iron, and manganese.

1 cup vegetable broth

¼ cup plus 1 tablespoon balsamic vinegar

¼ cup minced garlic

2 pounds (4 to 5 cups) Brussels sprouts, stems trimmed, any large sprouts halved lengthwise

3 tablespoons red pepper flakes (optional)

2 tablespoons garlic powder (optional)

Salt

1 Preheat the oven to 400°F.

2 In a large bowl, stir the vegetable broth together with the vinegar and garlic. Add the Brussels sprouts, and stir gently to coat.

3 Line a large, rimmed baking sheet with parchment paper or a silicone baking mat (or lightly spray the sheet with olive oil spray, but it will add a slight amount of fat). Spread the Brussels sprouts on the prepared sheet in a single layer.

| FB | | G-F | P | V |

PER SERVING

Calories **67.2** Carbohydrates **10.6g** Fat **1g** Protein **6.3g**   ½ cup

4 Sprinkle the Brussels sprouts generously with the red pepper flakes and garlic powder (if using), and season with salt. Bake for 25 to 35 minutes, until the Brussels sprouts are just tender.

5 Stir, sprinkle with more red pepper flakes and garlic powder (if using), and season again with salt. Bake for 15 to 25 minutes more, until the sprouts are tender when pierced with a sharp knife (cooking time will vary based on the size of the sprouts).

6 Transfer to a platter, plates, or meal prep containers, and serve hot or warm.

Time-saving tip: Before you dress the Brussels sprouts in the vegetable stock mixture, blanch them in a pot of boiling salted water for 10 to 15 minutes, or precook them in the microwave: Place them in a microwave-safe bowl with ½ cup of water and cover with plastic wrap. Cut a small slit in the plastic to allow steam to vent. Microwave on high for 10 minutes. Drain the Brussels sprouts, then proceed with the recipe. This will cut the overall cooking time by 15 to 20 minutes, depending on the size of your Brussels sprouts.

ZUCCHINI FRITTERS

MAKES 8 FRITTERS / PREP TIME: 15 MINUTES, PLUS 10 MINUTES TO STAND / COOK TIME: 10 MINUTES

Filling, low calorie, and full of healthy fats, these fritters make a great side dish, appetizer, or snack.

4 large zucchini

1 tablespoon salt

½ cup coconut or almond flour

1 tablespoon flaxseed meal

½ cup (4 or 5) egg whites

¼ cup chopped green onions

1 to 2 tablespoons coconut oil, as needed, divided

1 In a food processor fitted with the shredding disk, or using the large holes of a box grater, grate the zucchini. You should have 4 cups. Add the salt, and stir to mix. Transfer to a colander set over the sink, and let stand for 10 minutes.

2 Using your hands or a kitchen towel, squeeze the zucchini tightly to extract excess moisture (the drier the better).

3 Transfer the dried zucchini to a large mixing bowl, add the coconut flour, flaxseed meal, egg whites, and green onions, and mix well.

4 Press enough of the mixture firmly into a ½-cup measuring cup to fill the cup.

5 Heat half of the coconut oil in a pan with a lid large enough to fit four fritters over medium heat. Add the fritter from the measuring cup, make three more fritters, and add them to the pan. Cover, and cook for 2 to 3 minutes, until brown on the bottom.

6 Uncover, flip the fritters, cover again, and cook for another 2 to 3 minutes. The fritters should be brown on each side.

7 Serve warm.

Time-saving tip: You can leave any extra mixture in the fridge for a few days. That way you can fry them up fresh right before you enjoy them.

Serving tip: Try these fritters garnished with a dollop of Greek yogurt (remember to add the calories to the total).

FB **D-F** **G-F** **P**

PER SERVING

Calories **60** Carbohydrates **7.9g** Fat **3.2g** Protein **4.5g**

1 fritter

SAVORY ROASTED CAULIFLOWER

SERVES 3 / PREP TIME: 5 MINUTES / COOK TIME: 1 HOUR

Ideal for batch cooking

These little florets taste way too good to be this good for you. Savory spices give a deep, rich flavor that would complement any roast. A great substitute for potatoes and gravy, this superfood is superdelicious.

½ cup low-sodium vegetable broth

1 teaspoon ground cumin

1 teaspoon garlic powder

1 teaspoon nutritional yeast

1 teaspoon salt, plus more if desired

1 teaspoon freshly squeezed lime juice, plus more if desired

4 cups small cauliflower florets

Ingredient tip: *Nutritional yeast is available online, in the bulk food section of many grocery stores, or in some health food aisles.*

Time-saving tip: *After the florets are coated in the broth, cover the mixing bowl with plastic wrap. Poke one small slit to allow steam to vent. Microwave on high for 10 minutes. Proceed with the recipe from step 5, but only roast for 15 to 25 minutes, until tender. This will produce slightly softer cauliflower at the end, but it will be ready in less than half the time.*

1 Preheat the oven to 350°F.

2 In a large bowl, whisk the broth, cumin, garlic powder, nutritional yeast, salt, and lime juice until the spices are well blended and the salt is dissolved.

3 Add the cauliflower florets to the broth mixture, and toss to coat.

4 Line a rimmed baking sheet with parchment paper or a silicone baking mat (or lightly grease with extra-virgin olive oil spray, but this will add a slight amount of fat). Spread the cauliflower florets on the prepared sheet in a single layer.

5 Roast for 40 to 60 minutes, stirring occasionally, until the florets are tender.

6 Transfer the florets to plates or a platter, season with more lime juice and salt, if desired, and serve hot or warm.

	FB			G-F	P	V

PER SERVING

Calories **33** Carbohydrates **7g** Fat **0g** Protein **2.7g**

1 cup

PROTEIN MASHED POTATOES

MAKES 8 CUPS / PREP TIME: 10 MINUTES / COOK TIME: 10 MINUTES

Ideal for batch cooking • Ideal for post-workout

As creamy and tasty as mashed potatoes loaded with sour cream, these have the added protein (and zero fat) of Greek yogurt, plus heart-healthy fat from olive oil.

3 pounds russet potatoes, peeled and cut into 1-inch cubes

1 cup water, plus more for boiling

2 tablespoons salt, plus more for seasoning

1 cup nonfat Greek yogurt, divided

¼ cup plus 1 tablespoon extra-virgin olive oil

Freshly ground black pepper

Cooking tip: *Get creative and change up the flavor. Along with salt and pepper, stir in favorite herbs and spices like finely chopped garlic or chives.*

1 In a large pot, cover the potatoes with cold water, add the salt, and bring to a boil. Lower the heat, and simmer until the potatoes fall apart easily when pressed with a fork, about 10 minutes.

2 Meanwhile, in a medium bowl, whisk the 1 cup of water with ½ cup of yogurt until smooth (it should have the consistency of milk). Whisk in the olive oil, and set aside.

3 Drain the cooked potatoes, and transfer to a large bowl. Using a hand-held mixer on the lowest setting, or a masher, whisk, or with large fork, mash the potatoes. Gradually mix in just enough of the yogurt mixture so that the potatoes are creamy (you may not need all of the mixture).

4 Whisk in the remaining ½ cup of yogurt, season with salt and pepper, and serve hot.

MB   **G-F**

PER SERVING

Calories **132** Carbohydrates **19.8g** Fat **4.5g** Protein **3.8g**

½ cup

SAUTÉED RED CABBAGE
WITH HONEY AND MUSTARD SEEDS

MAKES 4 CUPS / PREP TIME: 5 MINUTES / COOK TIME: 15 MINUTES

Tangy-sweet and lightly crunchy, this easy side dish is overflowing with antioxidants and can be whipped up in minutes.

1 tablespoon extra-virgin olive oil

1 medium (about 4 ounces)
    red onion, sliced

12 cups (from 1 [2-pound] head)
    shredded red cabbage

½ cup apple cider vinegar

1 tablespoon honey

1½ teaspoons mustard seeds

Salt

Freshly ground black pepper

1 In a large skillet over medium-high heat, heat the olive oil. Add the red onion and cook, stirring often, until just softened, about 2 minutes.

2 Add the cabbage and cook, stirring gently, until wilted, about 4 minutes.

3 Sprinkle the vinegar over the cabbage, and stir gently to mix. Drizzle with the honey, sprinkle with the mustard seeds, and stir to combine. Reduce the heat to medium-low and cook, stirring occasionally, until the cabbage is tender, about 10 minutes more.

4 Season with salt and pepper, and serve hot or warm.

| FB | | | G-F | P | V |

PER SERVING

Calories **65** Carbohydrates **11.4g** Fat **1.9g** Protein **1.8g**

½ cup

FORBIDDEN FRIED RICE

MAKES 3 CUPS / PREP TIME: 5 MINUTES / COOK TIME: 30 MINUTES

Ideal for pre-workout • Ideal for batch cooking

Forbidden rice, also known as black rice, contains more antioxidants, iron, protein, and dietary fiber than any other kind of rice. You'll love its nutty flavor and chewy texture.

1 cup black or forbidden rice
2½ cups water, plus more for rinsing
   and more as needed
2 tablespoons coconut oil
3 green onions, chopped
1 tablespoon minced garlic
1 tablespoon ground ginger or
   3 tablespoons chopped fresh ginger
1 tablespoon red pepper flakes
4 cups baby spinach, chopped
Freshly squeezed lime juice,
   for garnish

1 Rinse the rice in several changes of cold tap water until the water runs clear.

2 In a large pot fitted with a lid, bring the 2½ cups of water to a boil. Stir in the rice, lower the heat to medium, and simmer uncovered for 30 minutes, stirring occasionally and adding more water as needed to keep the rice from scorching.

3 Cover the pot, remove from the heat, and let stand. You should have 3 cups of cooked rice.

4 In a large skillet over medium-high heat, heat the coconut oil. Add the green onions, garlic, ginger, and red pepper flakes, and cook, stirring, for 1 minute.

5 Stir in the cooked rice, and cook, stirring, for 1 minute more.

6 Add the spinach, and cook, stirring, until the spinach is wilted and the rice is crispy around the edges, about 1 minute more.

7 Remove from the heat, garnish with lime juice, and serve at once.

Cooking tip: *This dish can be cooked in bulk and refrigerated for up to 1 week.*

MB				G-F	P	V

PER SERVING   Calories **151** Carbohydrates **25g** Fat **5.5g** Protein **3.6g**   ½ cup

FUL MEDAMES

MAKES 5 CUPS / PREP TIME: 5 MINUTES / COOK TIME: 20 MINUTES

If you like hummus, you'll love this Middle-Eastern dip made from fava beans, one of the most nutritious beans. Fava beans' flavor is smoother, sweeter, and richer than most other beans. They offer just as much protein as other popular bean varieties, but are lower in calories. Serve this as a dip, too, with your favorite veggies.

Extra-virgin olive oil spray, if needed

1 medium yellow onion, chopped

2 teaspoons minced garlic

2 medium tomatoes, chopped,
   1 tablespoon reserved for garnish

3 cups canned fava beans, drained
   and rinsed

1 teaspoon ground cumin

¼ teaspoon ground cayenne pepper

3 tablespoons freshly squeezed
   lemon juice

Ingredient tip: Canned fava beans are also called broad beans. If your local store doesn't carry them, try online.

1 Heat a nonstick skillet over medium heat. If needed, lightly coat with olive oil spray to prevent sticking (this will add a slight amount of fat). Add the onion and garlic, and cook for 3 to 4 minutes, stirring occasionally, until just softened.

2 Add the tomatoes, and cook for 3 to 4 minutes, stirring occasionally, until heated through.

3 Add the fava beans, cumin, and cayenne pepper to the skillet. Turn the heat down to medium-low, and cook for 10 minutes, stirring occasionally, until slightly thickened.

4 Transfer the contents of the skillet to a serving bowl. Mash the fava beans with a fork to form a coarse puree, and stir in the lemon juice.

5 Garnish with the reserved tomato and serve.

MB   G-F   P   V

PER SERVING

Calories **107** Carbohydrate **11.6g** Fat **0.5g** Protein **6g**

1 cup

COLESLAW

MAKES 7 CUPS / PREP TIME: 10 MINUTES, PLUS 15 MINUTES TO STAND

Ideal for batch cooking

Traditional coleslaw is weighed down with calories from sugar and fat.
This leaner version is sweetened with stevia and lightly dressed with olive oil.
A great companion to any barbecue, this makes enough to feed a family—or to
provide one muscle-bound bodybuilder with days' worth of side dishes.

FOR THE SLAW

1 small head green cabbage
    (about 4 inches in diameter)

1 small head red cabbage
    (about 4 inches in diameter)

1 medium yellow onion

2 large carrots

⅓ cup salt

FOR THE DRESSING

1 cup apple cider vinegar

1 cup granulated stevia

2 tablespoons extra-virgin olive oil

1 teaspoon garlic powder

1 teaspoon freshly ground
    black pepper

1 teaspoon celery seeds

Salt, if needed

	FB		**LC**	**G-F**	**P**	**V**

PER SERVING · **1 cup**

Calories: **50**; Carbohydrates: **7.7g**; Fat: **2.2g**; Protein: **1.4g**

TO MAKE THE SLAW

1 Using a large, sharp knife, a mandoline, or a food processor fitted with the shredding disk, finely shred the cabbages and onion. Peel and grate the carrots.

2 In a large bowl, toss the cabbage, onion, and carrots with the salt. Let stand for at least 15 minutes, and up to 1 hour.

3 Transfer the cabbage mixture to a colander in the sink, and rinse thoroughly under cold running water to remove the salt. If the cabbage mixture seems soggy, transfer to a paper towel–lined baking sheet and pat dry (the less soggy the cabbage, the better the slaw).

TO MAKE THE DRESSING

1 In a large, clean bowl, whisk the apple cider vinegar, stevia, olive oil, garlic powder, pepper, and celery seeds.

2 Add the cabbage mixture, and toss to coat. Season with more salt, pepper, and stevia if needed, and serve.

QUINOA
WITH MUSHROOMS AND SPINACH

MAKES 5 CUPS / PREP TIME: 10 MINUTES / COOK TIME: 20 MINUTES

Ideal for pre-workout

This savory side is a nice balance of protein, carbs, and fiber. The spinach and vitamin–D rich mushrooms give the quinoa even more muscle-building and fat-burning power.

3 teaspoons extra-virgin olive oil, divided

1 medium (about 4 ounces) yellow onion, chopped

1 teaspoon minced garlic

1 cup quinoa

2½ cups low-sodium vegetable broth, divided

2 tablespoons balsamic vinegar, divided

2 teaspoons chopped fresh thyme leaves, divided

8 ounces mushrooms, sliced

10 ounces baby spinach leaves

Salt

Freshly ground black pepper

1 In a large saucepan over medium-high heat, heat 1½ teaspoons of olive oil. Add the onion and garlic, and cook, stirring, for about 5 minutes, until the onion has softened and turned translucent. Stir in the quinoa.

2 Add 2 cups of broth, 2 teaspoons of balsamic vinegar, and 1 teaspoon of thyme.

3 Bring to a boil, reduce the heat to medium-low, cover, and simmer for about 15 minutes, until the quinoa is tender.

MB

G-F **P** **V**

PER SERVING

Calories **200** Carbohydrates **32g** Fat **4.6g** Protein **7.8g**

1 cup

4 Meanwhile, in a large skillet over medium-high heat, heat the remaining 1½ teaspoons of olive oil. Add the mushrooms, and cook for about 5 minutes, stirring often, until lightly browned.

5 Add the remaining ½ cup of vegetable broth, the remaining 4 teaspoons of balsamic vinegar, and the remaining 1 teaspoon of chopped thyme to the mushrooms, and stir to coat. Reduce the heat to medium-low, cover, and simmer for about 5 minutes, until the mushrooms have softened.

6 When the quinoa has cooked, add the mushroom mixture to the saucepan and mix well.

7 Remove the quinoa from the heat, and immediately fold in the spinach leaves (do this quickly while the quinoa is still hot to ensure the spinach wilts completely).

8 Season with salt and pepper and serve hot or warm.

ROASTED SWEETS AND BEETS

MAKES 5 SERVINGS / PREP TIME: 10 MINUTES / COOKING TIME: 45 MINUTES

Ideal for pre-workout • Ideal for batch cooking

Sweet and salty, this colorful side dish is a tasty treat packed with beta-carotene-loaded sweet potatoes and performance-enhancing beets. Put it in your weekly meal prep, or impress your guests at your next holiday dinner with this beautiful side dish.

2 (15-ounce) cans small whole beets, rinsed and quartered

1 pound sweet potatoes, peeled if you prefer, cut into ½-inch chunks

1 large Vidalia onion or Walla Walla onion, chopped

1 tablespoon extra-virgin olive oil

1 teaspoon garlic powder

1 teaspoon salt

1 teaspoon freshly ground black pepper

1 Preheat the oven to 400°F.

2 In a large bowl, toss the beets, sweet potatoes, onion, olive oil, garlic, salt, and pepper. Spread in a single layer on a foil-lined baking sheet.

3 Bake for 30 to 45 minutes, stirring halfway, until the sweet potatoes are tender.

4 Serve warm or hot.

Cooking tip: *The oven temperature is flexible. If you are roasting or baking something else at a different temperature, feel free to throw the sweet potatoes in alongside it. Lower temperatures will increase the total cooking time.*

Ingredient tip: *You can use fresh beets rather than canned, if you prefer.*

MB			G-F	P	V

PER SERVING

Calories **149** Carbohydrates **29.2g** Fat **3g** Protein **2.6g**

CHUNKY APPLESAUCE

MAKES 3 CUPS / PREP TIME: 5 MINUTES / COOK TIME: 15 MINUTES

Ideal for post-workout

A tasty way to eat your apples, and the perfect side dish for pork or a pre- or post-workout snack.

2 large apples

1½ teaspoons coconut oil

3 tablespoons water

1 tablespoon ground cinnamon (optional), plus more for seasoning

1 teaspoon freshly squeezed lemon juice

1 to 2 tablespoons granulated stevia (optional)

1 Core the apples, and cut them into small chunks (do not peel them). The smaller the chunks, the faster the sauce will cook.

2 In a large skillet over medium-high heat, melt the coconut oil. Add the apple chunks, and stir to coat them with the oil.

3 Sprinkle the apples with the water, cinnamon (if using), and lemon juice. Cover and cook, stirring occasionally, until the apples are tender, 10 to 15 minutes, depending on the size of your chunks.

4 Season with more cinnamon and stevia, if desired, and serve warm or cold.

Cooking tip: *You can use pretty much any apple here. Sweeter varieties make for a sweeter sauce.*

MB			G-F	P	V

PER SERVING

Calories **50** Carbohydrates **10.3g** Fat **1.3g** Protein **0.2g**

½ cup

STIR-FRIED BROCCOLI
WITH GARLIC

MAKES 8 CUPS / PREP TIME: 3 MINUTES / COOK TIME: 10 MINUTES

Ideal for batch cooking

Chinese take-out doesn't hold a candle to this amazing side dish. It has all the healthy benefits of broccoli with a delicious Asian spin. Easy to make at home in minutes, this is a great companion to any Asian-inspired main course.

1 cup low-sodium vegetable broth

¼ cup gluten-free soy sauce or liquid aminos

2 tablespoons cornstarch

3 teaspoons minced garlic

3 tablespoons sesame oil

8 cups (from 2 large heads) broccoli florets

Red pepper flakes (optional)

1 In a small bowl, whisk the vegetable broth with the soy sauce, cornstarch, and garlic. Set the sauce aside.

2 In a large skillet over medium-high heat, heat the sesame oil. Add the broccoli florets, and cook, stirring frequently, until tender, about 5 minutes.

3 Reduce the heat to medium-low, add the reserved sauce, and stir well to coat.

4 Cook for about 3 more minutes, stirring a few times, until the sauce has thickened, and serve.

Cooking tip: *If you prefer more tender broccoli, steam the florets in the microwave or on the stove for a few minutes before adding them to the skillet.*

| FB | | G-F | P | V |

PER SERVING

Calories **50** Carbohydrates **7.7g** Fat **2.2g** Protein **1.4g**

1 cup

BEETS AND GREEN BEANS

MAKES 4½ CUPS / PREP TIME: 15 MINUTES / COOK TIME: 20 MINUTES

Ideal for pre-workout • Ideal for batch cooking

This tangy, colorful beet-and-bean medley is full of flavor, fiber, and endurance-boosting nutrients. A great side dish to any grilled or baked meat entrée.

1 tablespoon extra-virgin olive oil

1 medium (about 4 ounces)
  red onion, chopped

4 cups green beans, trimmed and cut
  into 2-inch pieces

½ cup water

3 tablespoons apple cider vinegar

1 tablespoon minced garlic

1 teaspoon dried thyme or 8 sprigs
  fresh thyme, chopped

½ teaspoon red pepper flakes

1 cup canned whole beets or baked
  fresh beets, cut into ½-inch cubes

1 large tomato, chopped

Salt

Freshly ground black pepper

1 In a large skillet over medium-high heat, heat the olive oil. Add the onion and beans, and cook for about 10 minutes, stirring frequently, until the onion is transparent.

2 Add the water, cover, and cook for 5 minutes more.

3 Add the apple cider vinegar, garlic, thyme, and red pepper, and mix.

4 Add the beets and tomato, folding them gently into the beans. Continue cooking until the beets are heated through, about 5 more minutes. Season with salt and pepper and serve.

Ingredient tip: *To bake the beets, slice off the leaves close to their tips. Wash the beets thoroughly, and wrap each loosely in foil. Roast in a 400°F oven for about 1 hour, checking every 15 minutes. If they seem dry or the bottoms are scorching, add a little water to each beet, rewrap, and continue roasting. They are ready when easily pierced with a fork in the center. Cool the beets and peel.*

| FB | | LC | G-F | P | V |

PER SERVING

Calories **46** Carbohydrates **7.3g** Fat **1.7g** Protein **1.5g**

½ cup

SWEET POTATO FRIES
WITH ROSEMARY

SERVES 5 / PREP TIME: 15 MINUTES / COOK TIME: 30 MINUTES

Make these delicate and delightful restaurant-quality sweet potato fries right in your own kitchen, with way less fat and salt. Crispy on the outside and tender on the inside, these fries have just the right amount of rosemary to enhance their flavor.

1 pound sweet potatoes
2 tablespoons extra-virgin olive oil, divided
1 tablespoon chopped fresh rosemary (optional but recommended)
Salt

1 Preheat the oven to 450°F.

2 Line two rimmed baking sheets with parchment paper or a silicone baking mat (or lightly coat with extra-virgin olive oil spray, but this will add a slight amount of fat).

3 Peel the sweet potatoes, but do not rinse them (you need them dry so the oil adheres).

4 Using a sharp knife or a mandoline fitted with the julienne attachment, cut the sweet potatoes into ½-inch-thick fries.

5 Transfer the sweet potato fries to a large bowl, and drizzle in the olive oil 2 teaspoons at a time, tossing to coat. You may not need all of the oil; the fries should be evenly coated and shiny but not dripping.

6 Spread the fries onto the prepared baking sheets in a single layer, without crowding. No fries should be touching. Use additional baking sheets if needed.

7 Sprinkle the fries with the rosemary and salt, and bake for 15 minutes.

8 Using a spatula or tongs, flip the fries over. Continue baking for 10 to 15 minutes longer, until the fries are golden and crispy.

9 Divide into five equal servings, and serve warm.

MB				G-F	P	V

PER SERVING

Calories **125** Carbohydrates **18.2g** Fat **5.4g** Protein **1.4g**

3.2 ounces

CREAMY CUCUMBER SALAD

MAKES 6 CUPS /
PREP TIME: 15 MINUTES, PLUS 30 MINUTES TO STAND AND 30 MINUTES TO CHILL

A healthy twist on Greek tzatziki, this refreshing side dish is pumped up with protein-packed nonfat Greek yogurt. It's a perfect companion to fish and a winning addition to a summer barbecue.

3 medium cucumbers
   (about 1½ pounds total)
2 tablespoons salt, plus more
   for seasoning
1 medium (about 4 ounces) white
   onion, quartered
1 cup nonfat Greek yogurt
Freshly ground black pepper
Ground smoked paprika or chopped
   fresh dill weed, for garnish

1 Using a sharp knife, cut off and discard the ends of the cucumbers. Cut off a small slice of each cucumber, and taste it for bitterness. If the cucumber tastes bitter, remove the peel. If the taste is pleasant, leave the skin on. Using a mandoline or a sharp knife, thinly slice the cucumbers (the thinner the better).

2 Transfer the cucumbers to a colander set in the sink, sprinkle with the 2 tablespoons of salt, and toss to coat. Let stand for at least 30 minutes to draw out excess moisture.

3 Meanwhile, using the mandoline or sharp knife, slice each onion quarter as thinly as possible.

4 Using your hands or kitchen towels, squeeze the cucumbers to remove as much moisture as possible.

5 In a serving bowl, toss the cucumbers and onion with the yogurt. Season with salt and pepper.

6 Cover and refrigerate for at least 30 minutes, preferably overnight or more. The longer the cucumbers marinate, the better the flavor.

7 Sprinkle with paprika or dill and serve.

FB   **LC**   **G-F**

PER SERVING

Calories **44** Carbohydrates **7g** Fat **0g** Protein **4.7g**

1 cup

SPINACH AND SPAGHETTI SQUASH SOUFFLÉ

**MAKES 8 SLICES / PREP TIME: 5 MINUTES /
COOK TIME: 45 MINUTES / TOTAL TIME: 1 HOUR**

This low-fat, low-calorie veggie-filled soufflé showcases spaghetti squash's mild flavor and tender texture, which provides most of the soufflé's volume. The squash and spinach meld with the mozzarella to make a delicious addition to any table.

Extra-virgin olive oil spray

1 cup (1½ medium) chopped onion

1 cup chopped baby kale

3 cups (1 [5-ounce] bag) baby spinach

2 cups baked spaghetti squash,
   drained of extra liquid

4 egg whites

2 eggs

½ cup shredded nonfat mozzarella

2 tablespoons nutritional yeast

1 teaspoon sea salt

1 teaspoon freshly ground
   black pepper

Ingredient tips: Nutritional yeast is available online, in the bulk food section of many grocery stores, or in some health food aisles.

To easily bake the spaghetti squash, cut in half lengthwise, scoop out the seeds, and bake in the microwave for about 15 minutes or in a 350°F oven for about 40 minutes, until the skin can easily be poked with a fork. Make sure the baked and cooled squash is well drained so the quiche doesn't get runny.

FB **D-F** **G-F**

PER SERVING

Calories **59** Carbohydrates **5.3g** Fat **2.8g** Protein **6.7g**

1 slice

1 Preheat the oven to 350°F.

2 Heat a medium skillet over medium-high heat, and lightly coat with olive oil spray. Add the onion, and cook for about 5 minutes, until tender. Add the kale and spinach, and cook for about 3 minutes, until the kale is tender and the spinach is wilted. Remove from the heat.

3 In a medium bowl, use a fork to mix the spaghetti squash, cooked vegetables, egg whites, eggs, mozzarella, nutritional yeast, salt, and black pepper until the eggs are beaten and all the ingredients are well mixed.

4 Lightly coat a 9-inch pie dish with olive oil spray. Pour the mixture into the pie dish, and bake for 35 minutes, until the top is golden and the eggs are firmly set.

5 Let rest for 10 minutes, cut into 8 slices, and serve warm. Leftovers can be stored in a tightly sealed container in the fridge for up to one week.

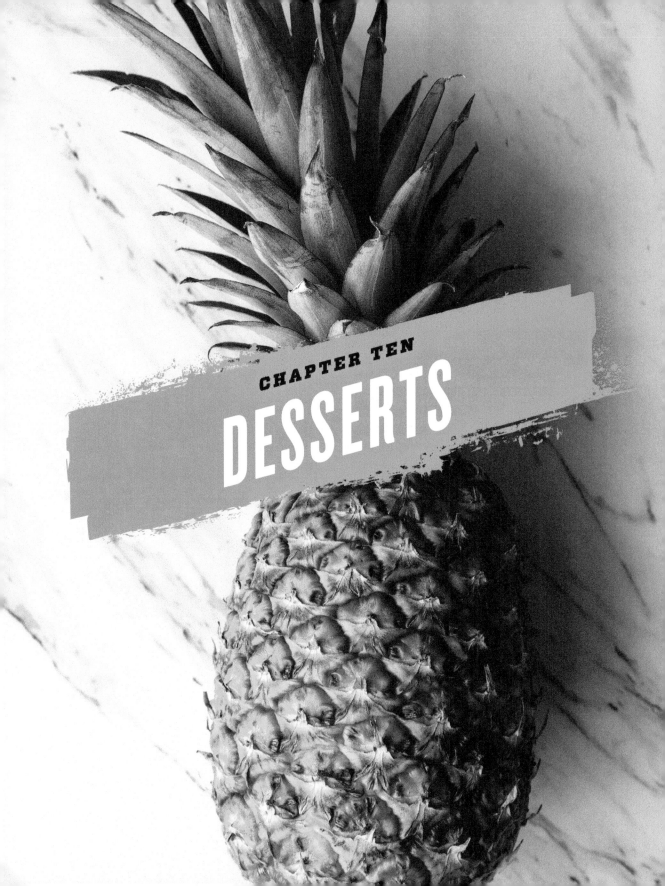

CHAPTER TEN

DESSERTS

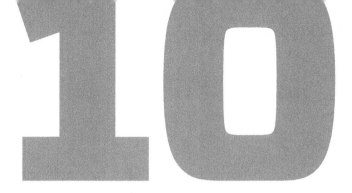

Your craving for sweets doesn't have to send you spiraling off your diet. Each of the recipes in this chapter will hit your sweet spot without breaking your calorie budget. With some simple substitutions, they offer delicious and nutritious ways to enjoy dessert. Traditional dessert recipes provide very little nutritional value considering the large number of calories per serving. All the fats and carbohydrates here come from healthy sources packed with nutrients, and many are beefed up with muscle-building protein as well. After all the hard work you're putting in at the gym, you deserve to treat yourself a little, so go ahead and enjoy!

MB Muscle Building **FB** Fat Burning **D-F** Dairy-Free **LC** Low Carb **G-F** Gluten-Free **P** Paleo **V** Vegan

RASPBERRY SORBET

SERVES 1 / PREP TIME: 3 MINUTES

Ideal for post-workout

This refreshing treat can be whipped up in minutes, and makes the perfect dessert or sweet little snack. It's low in calories and packed with flavor, and it's easy to make just a single serving—or you can up the ingredients to satisfy a group of friends.

1 cup frozen raspberries
½ cup sugar-free vanilla almond milk
¼ cup granulated stevia

1 In a food processor or blender, blend the raspberries, almond milk, and stevia until a thick, smooth texture is formed. You will have to shake or stir the ingredients a few times. Avoid the urge to add extra almond milk. It will make the sorbet runny.

2 Spoon into a serving bowl and enjoy.

Time-saving tip: *This sorbet can be prepared in advance and stored in the freezer for several hours. If it freezes solid, rest in the refrigerator to soften.*

FB　　　**G-F**　**P**

PER SERVING

Calories **85**　Carbohydrates **17g**　Fat **2g**　Protein **2g**

CHOCOLATE-CHIA MOUSSE

**SERVES 8 / PREP TIME: 10 MINUTES, PLUS 5 MINUTES TO SOAK /
COOK TIME: 45 MINUTES / TOTAL TIME: 1 HOUR, 30 MINUTES**

A great way to enjoy your healthy fats, this silky smooth mousse with lush avocado and fiber-rich chia seeds is just delicious.

2 tablespoons chia seeds

½ cup water

1 avocado

6 tablespoons unsweetened
   cocoa powder

1 teaspoon vanilla extract

6 egg whites

¼ teaspoon cream of tartar

1 cup granulated stevia, plus more
   for serving

Fresh fruit, for serving (optional)

Ground cinnamon, for serving (optional)

1 Preheat the oven to 350°F.

2 In a small bowl, soak the chia seeds in the water for about 5 minutes, until they form a gel.

3 In a food processor or blender, blend the chia gel, avocado, cocoa powder, and vanilla until smooth.

4 In a large bowl, whip the egg whites and cream of tartar until stiff peaks form. Gradually add the stevia and the chia–cocoa powder mixture.

5 Pour into 8 ramekins or a baking-cup-lined muffin tin. Place in a water bath (a larger pan filled with water), and bake for 45 minutes.

6 The center will still be gooey. Transfer to the refrigerator for about 30 minutes to chill completely.

7 To serve, top with some fresh fruit or sprinkle with cinnamon and a little more stevia (remember to add calories from the fruit to the total).

MB   **D-F**   **LC**   **G-F**   **P**

PER SERVING

Calories **70** Carbohydrates **5.1g** Fat **4.4g** Protein **4.5g**

1 dish

GREEK YOGURT "CHEESECAKE"
WITH CHOCOLATE PROTEIN CRUMB CRUST

**MAKES 1 (8-BY-8-INCH) CAKE (SERVES 9) / PREP TIME: 10 MINUTES /
COOK TIME: 50 MINUTES / TOTAL TIME: 1 HOUR, 30 MINUTES**

Now you can have your cheese cake and eat it too, thanks to this truly guilt-free cheesecake packed with protein and good fats.

FOR THE CRUST

¼ cup almond flour

½ cup chocolate whey protein isolate

¼ cup unsweetened cocoa powder

3 tablespoons milled flaxseed

¼ cup granulated stevia or Splenda

3 tablespoons coconut oil, melted

Ingredient tip: If you don't have almond flour on hand, you can make your own by grinding up whole almonds in a blender until they form a flour.

FOR THE FILLING

2 eggs

2 cups nonfat Greek yogurt

1 teaspoon vanilla

½ cup granulated stevia

1 tablespoon gluten-free all-purpose baking mix

Sugar-free jelly, for serving (optional)

FB **LC** **G-F**

PER SERVING

Calories **145** Carbohydrates **5.9g** Fat **8.8g** Protein **13.2g**

1 slice

Preheat the oven to 300°F.

TO MAKE THE CRUST

1 In a medium bowl, mix the almond flour, whey protein, cocoa powder, flaxseed, and stevia. Gradually add the melted coconut oil, and mix until large crumbs form.

2 Transfer to an ungreased 8-by-8-inch pan, spreading over the bottom and pressing the crumb mixture firmly down to form an even crust.

TO MAKE THE FILLING

1 In a medium bowl, beat the eggs. Add the yogurt, and mix until smooth. Add the vanilla, and then gradually stir in the stevia and baking mix. Pour the mixture into the crust.

2 Bake for 45 to 50 minutes, until the center is firm.

3 Allow to cool completely, about 30 minutes.

4 Cut into nine even slices and serve plain or with a sugar-free jelly (remember to add the calories from the jelly to the total).

PERFECT PUMPKIN PIE

MAKES 1 (9-INCH) PIE (SERVES 8) / PREP TIME: 20 MINUTES /
COOK TIME: 35 MINUTES / TOTAL TIME: 1 HOUR, 25 MINUTES

This fall favorite you can finally feel good about is packed with fiber, protein,
and fat-burning spices.

FOR THE CRUST

2 tablespoons psyllium husk

⅛ teaspoon xanthan gum

⅓ cup hot water

1¼ cups almond flour

½ cup unsalted raw almonds

½ cup cornstarch

⅛ teaspoon salt

½ teaspoon baking soda

3 to 4 tablespoons water, if needed

Coconut oil, for greasing

FOR THE FILLING

1 (15-ounce) can 100% pure pumpkin

½ cup nonfat Greek yogurt

1 cup fat-free cottage cheese

1 cup (from 8 to 12 eggs) egg whites

3 teaspoons ground cinnamon

1 teaspoon ground allspice

1 teaspoon ground ginger

1 teaspoon ground nutmeg

½ teaspoon ground cloves

½ teaspoon salt

1 cup granulated stevia

MB　　　　　　**G-F**

PER SERVING

Calories **215** Carbohydrates **18g** Fat **10.7g** Protein **12.9g**

1 slice

Preheat the oven to 300°F.

TO MAKE THE CRUST

1 In a small bowl, mix the psyllium husk, xanthan gum, and hot water. Allow the mixture to sit and thicken for 5 minutes.

2 Meanwhile, in a blender or food processor, process the almond flour, almonds, cornstarch, salt, and baking soda, stopping to stir and scrape down the sides as needed, until a fine flour forms.

3 Add the psyllium husk mixture to the food processor, and process. If the dough is still crumbly, add 1 tablespoon of water at a time, blending between additions, until the dough clumps together.

4 Place the dough on a piece of parchment paper or a silicone baking sheet, and roll into a 10-inch circle.

5 Place the dough in a lightly greased 9-inch pie tin using this easy trick with 2 pie tins: First, place 1 pie tin upside down on your work surface. Pick up the parchment paper with the dough, and drape it dough-side-down onto the overturned pie tin. Peel off the parchment paper, and place the second pie tin over the dough. Flip the whole thing over, and remove the inner pie tin. This may seem like extra work, but it does a great job of preventing rips or tears in the dough.

TO MAKE THE FILLING

1 In a blender or food processor, blend the pumpkin, yogurt, cottage cheese, egg whites, cinnamon, allspice, ginger, nutmeg, cloves, salt, and stevia on high for 2 to 3 minutes, until smooth. Pour the mixture over the crust.

2 Bake for 25 to 35 minutes, until small cracks start to form on the filling. If you gently shake the pie, the filling will still wiggle.

3 Remove the pie from the oven, and allow it to cool completely, about 30 minutes.

4 Cut into eight even slices and serve.

SUGAR- AND GLUTEN-FREE PEANUT BUTTER COOKIES

MAKES 16 COOKIES / PREP TIME: 10 MINUTES / COOK TIME: 10 MINUTES

Cookies and healthy fats in your diet? Yes! Of course, as with all healthy fats, they are nutrient-dense and have calories equivalent to the fats they provide, so watch your portions. You can add a serving of nuts, too, and not throw off your macros.

1 egg white
1 tablespoon vanilla extract
1 tablespoon milled flaxseed
1 cup natural creamy peanut butter
1 cup granulated stevia

1 Preheat the oven to 350°F.

2 Line a cookie sheet with parchment paper or a silicone baking sheet.

3 In a small bowl, mix the egg white, vanilla, and flaxseed. Set aside to rest.

4 If any oil has separated from the peanut butter, mix together until smooth. In a large bowl, mix the peanut butter and stevia. Add the egg white mixture, and mix until smooth with no visible stevia granules.

5 Scoop out about 1 tablespoon of dough, and roll it into a ball; you should have about 16 even balls. Place the balls on the prepared sheet. Using a fork, make a crosshatch by gently pressing down in one direction, then again in another, making the crisscross pattern.

6 Bake for 8 to 12 minutes. Less time will give a softer cookie, more time will give a crispier cookie.

7 Cool for a few minutes before removing the cookies from the baking sheet and serving.

Ingredient tip: *Use a natural peanut butter. The only ingredients should be dry-roasted peanuts and salt, if it is salted. Salted peanut butter will give a saltier cookie, unsalted a sweeter cookie.*

MB		LC	G-F	P	V

PER SERVING

Calories **98** Carbohydrates **3.6g** Fat **8g** Protein **4.3g**

1 cookie

PROTEIN PUMPKIN-SPICE COOKIES

**MAKES 30 COOKIES / PREP TIME: 10 MINUTES /
COOK TIME: 10 MINUTES / TOTAL TIME: 35 MINUTES**

The delicious flavor of a pumpkin pie in a healthy protein powder–based cookie, these cookies turn out delicious in just minutes.

3 scoops whey protein isolate powder, vanilla or cinnamon flavor

1 cup granulated stevia

2 teaspoons ground cinnamon

1 teaspoon ground nutmeg

½ teaspoon ground allspice

½ teaspoon baking powder

½ teaspoon baking soda

1 scoop casein protein powder, vanilla or cinnamon flavor

½ cup water

2 egg whites

1 tablespoon coconut oil, melted

1 cup 100% pure canned pumpkin

1 Preheat the oven to 350°F.

2 In a large bowl, mix the whey, stevia, cinnamon, nutmeg, allspice, baking powder, and baking soda.

3 In a medium bowl, stir the casein and water well. Stir in the egg whites, coconut oil, and pumpkin.

4 Add the wet ingredients to the dry, and mix together.

5 Spoon the dough onto a lightly greased cookie sheet to form about 30 cookies.

6 Bake for 6 to 8 minutes. Cool completely, about 15 minutes, and then use a spatula to remove from the baking sheet.

Ingredient tip: Not all protein powders are created equal. Choose wisely to ensure the best texture and flavor.

FB **LC** **G-F**

PER SERVING

Calories **25** Carbohydrates **1.2g** Fat **0.6g** Protein **4.2g**

1 cookie

APPLE PIE POCKETS

**SERVES 12 / PREP TIME: 25 MINUTES / COOK TIME: 20 MINUTES /
TOTAL TIME: 55 MINUTES**

Ideal for post-workout • Ideal for batch cooking

These Apple Pie Pockets make a great dessert or grab-and-go snack. Though gluten-free, the texture of the dough is exactly like a regular pie crust, and the apple filling provides a naturally sweet center. A great source of fiber and healthy fats with all the muscle-building and fat-burning elements of apples.

FOR THE CRUST

2 tablespoons psyllium husk

⅛ teaspoon xanthan gum

⅓ cup hot water

1¼ cups almond flour

½ cup unsalted raw almonds

½ cup cornstarch

⅛ teaspoon salt

½ teaspoon baking soda

3 to 4 tablespoons water, if needed

FOR THE FILLING

3 cups (6 medium) finely chopped
   Granny Smith apples

2 tablespoons ground cinnamon

½ cup granulated stevia, or as desired

Preheat the oven to 350°F.

TO MAKE THE CRUST

1 In a small bowl, mix the psyllium husk, xanthan gum, and hot water. Set aside to thicken into a gel.

2 In a food processor or blender, process the almond flour, almonds, cornstarch, salt, and baking soda, stopping to stir and scrape down the sides as needed, until a fine flour forms.

3 Add the psyllium husk gel mixture to the food processor, and process. If the dough is still crumbly, add 1 tablespoon of water at a time, blending between additions, until the dough clumps together.

MB **G-F** **V**

Calories **118** Carbohydrates **12.7g** Fat **7g** Protein **3.2g**

1 piece

4 Place the dough on a piece of parchment paper or a silicone baking sheet, roll it out into a thin even rectangle, and set aside.

TO MAKE THE FILLING

1 In a large bowl, mix the apples, cinnamon, and stevia.

2 Spread the apple filling on the dough, leaving a 1-inch border around the edges. Fold in the short edges of the rectangle. Fold the long edges in and over all the filling so that they meet in the center. Smooth out the dough to seal in the filling. It is okay to leave a short slit down the center where the dough meets to expose a small strip of filling, but try to eliminate any gaps or holes elsewhere.

3 Bake for 20 to 22 minutes, until the crust feels solid to the touch and the apples are bubbling through the slit. Note that the crust will not brown as it would with wheat flour.

4 Cool for at least 10 minutes. Cut in half down the length and into 6 down the width, forming 12 equal pieces. Store in the refrigerator for up to a week. Enjoy warm, cold, or at room temperature.

COCONUT MACAROONS

**MAKES 16 MACAROONS / PREP TIME: 15 MINUTES /
COOK TIME: 20 MINUTES / TOTAL TIME: 40 MINUTES**

These macaroons could not be easier to make! What a delicious way to work the super-healthy benefits of coconut into your diet.

3 egg whites

½ cup granulated stevia

1½ teaspoons vanilla extract

¼ teaspoon salt

2 cups reduced-fat unsweetened coconut flakes or shredded coconut

Ingredient tips: Unsweetened coconut flakes of normal fat content also work great. This will obviously raise the fat and calorie content slightly, but it is still all healthy fat. You can also use shredded coconut instead of coconut flakes. Shredded coconut will have finer coconut pieces, giving the macaroons a softer consistency. Flakes will come in larger pieces and be a bit chewier.

Use egg whites from whole eggs. They will hold the macaroons together better than pasteurized egg whites in a carton.

MB **D-F** **LC** **G-F** **P**

PER SERVING

Calories **38** Carbohydrates **2g** Fat **3g** Protein **1.2g**

1 macaroon

1 Preheat the oven to 325°F.

2 Line a baking sheet with parchment paper or a silicone baking mat.

3 In a medium bowl, whisk the egg whites until foamy.

4 Add the stevia, vanilla extract, and salt, and whisk well.

5 Put the coconut flakes in a medium bowl. Add the egg white mixture, a little at a time, to the coconut flakes. You may not need all of the mixture. You want to add just enough to hold the flakes together, but not so much that the egg white mixture is pooling in the bottom of the bowl. The macaroon mixture should feel a little sticky, making it possible to shape the macaroons.

6 With wet hands, make 16 balls (about the size of golf balls) from the coconut mixture, and place them on the prepared baking sheet.

7 Bake for 15 to 20 minutes, until some of the flakes look toasted and are no longer sticky to the touch.

8 Cool for 5 minutes and serve or store in an airtight container for up to a week.

KEY LIME PROTEIN PIE

**MAKES 1 PIE (SERVES 8) / PREP TIME: 20 MINUTES /
COOK TIME: 45 MINUTES / TOTAL TIME: 1 HOUR, 35 MINUTES**

This pie has all the tangy sweetness of key lime pie packed with protein, fiber, and fat-burning nutrients. You can feel good about eating this renovated version of a classic dessert.

FOR THE FILLING

2 egg whites

2 cups nonfat Greek yogurt

¾ cup granulated stevia

½ cup freshly squeezed key lime juice

1 teaspoon xanthan gum

1 tablespoon cornstarch

FOR THE CRUST

1 tablespoon milled flaxseed

4 tablespoons water

1 scoop whey isolate protein powder, vanilla or cinnamon flavor

¼ cup granulated stevia

¼ cup almond flour

1 teaspoon ground cinnamon

Extra-virgin olive oil spray

Preheat the oven to 300°F.

TO MAKE THE FILLING

1 In a large bowl, whisk the egg whites and Greek yogurt. Add the stevia, and mix well.

2 In a small microwave-safe bowl, heat the key lime juice in the microwave for 1½ to 2 minutes, until very hot. Stir in the xanthan gum, and mix until it dissolves completely. As the mixture cools, it should start to thicken. Once the key lime mixture is cool to touch, add it to the Greek yogurt mixture and stir.

3 Gradually add the cornstarch, mixing thoroughly between additions. Set the filling aside.

FB   **LC**   **G-F**

PER SERVING

Calories **100** Carbohydrates **6.3g** Fat **2.4g** Protein **14g**

1 slice

TO MAKE THE CRUST

1 In a small bowl, mix the flaxseed with the water, and set aside to thicken.

2 In a large bowl, mix the protein powder, stevia, almond flour, and cinnamon.

3 Gradually add the flaxseed mixture, and knead into a dough.

4 Lightly coat a pie tin with olive oil spray, and press the dough into the pie tin.

5 Pour the filling on top of the crust. Bake for 40 to 45 minutes, until the center is set and does not wiggle when you shake the pie tin and the top has browned slightly.

6 Transfer to the refrigerator to cool, about 30 minutes.

7 Cut into eight equal slices and serve cold.

Ingredient tip: *Not all protein powders are created equal. Choose wisely to ensure the best texture and flavor.*

PROTEIN PINEAPPLE JELL-O DESSERT

MAKES 6½ CUPS / PREP TIME: 10 MINUTES, PLUS 4 HOURS TO CHILL

Ideal for post-workout

This dessert has plenty of protein and just enough pineapple for a little pick-me-up. For extra post-workout carbs, top with some additional fresh pineapple.

2 cups nonfat Greek yogurt

3 scoops whey protein isolate, vanilla flavor

1 cup canned crushed pineapple in 100% pineapple juice, drained, plus more for serving, if desired

2 cups water

2 packets sugar free Jell-O, strawberry or lime flavor

Ingredient tip: *Not all protein powders are created equal. Choose wisely to ensure the best texture and flavor.*

1 In a large bowl, mix the yogurt, whey protein powder, and pineapple.

2 In a small microwaveable bowl, microwave the water for 5 minutes, or boil on the stove top. Immediately add the Jell-O, and stir until the powder is completely dissolved.

3 Stir the Jell-O into the yogurt mixture.

4 Refrigerate until solid, 4 hours and up to overnight. If you like, before refrigerating, transfer the mixture into a Jell-O mold that has been lightly coated with olive oil spray (this will add a slightly amount of fat). If using a mold, invert it, remove the center piece to release the Jell-O, and remove the lid.

5 Serve plain or topped with additional crushed pineapple (remember to add the extra calories to the total).

MB **LC** **G-F**

PER SERVING

Calories **69** Carbohydrates **6.5g** Fat **0.6g** Protein **9.2g**

½ cup

GERMAN CHOCOLATE– BLACK BEAN CAKE

**MAKES 1 (8-BY-8-INCH) CAKE (SERVES 8) / PREP TIME: 10 MINUTES /
COOK TIME: 15 MINUTES / TOTAL TIME: 40 MINUTES**

Ideal for post-workout

A soft, rich, and chocolaty cake so good you won't even want to frost it. You would never know a cake this amazing was made from black beans.

1 (15-ounce) can no-salt-added black beans, drained and rinsed

1 scoop whey isolate protein powder, chocolate flavor

⅓ cup honey or agave syrup

3 tablespoons coconut oil or canola oil

3 tablespoons natural unsweetened cocoa powder

2 tablespoons granulated stevia

1 tablespoon vanilla extract

½ teaspoon ground cinnamon

½ teaspoon baking soda

¼ teaspoon salt

⅓ cup chocolate chips

Extra-virgin olive oil spray

1 Preheat the oven to 350°F.

2 In a food processor or blender, process the black beans, protein powder, honey, coconut oil, cocoa powder, stevia, vanilla extract, cinnamon, baking soda, and salt until very smooth. Fold in the chocolate chips using a spoon.

3 Lightly coat an 8-by-8-inch baking dish with olive oil spray, and transfer the batter to the baking dish.

4 Bake for 15 minutes (the center may still seem a bit undone), and refrigerate immediately for 15 minutes to cool and set.

5 Cut into 8 bars, each about 4 by 2 inches, and serve or store covered in the refrigerator for up to a week.

MB   **D-F**   **G-F**

PER SERVING

Calories: **199**; Carbohydrates: **28.9g**; Fat: **8.25g**; Protein: **11g**

1 bar

CHOCOLATE PROTEIN MUG CAKE
WITH WHIPPED PEANUT BUTTER FROSTING

**MAKES 1 MUG CAKE (4 PIECES) / PREP TIME: 10 MINUTES /
COOKING TIME: 3 MINUTES / TOTAL TIME: 23 MINUTES**

This protein cake tastes as good as any gluten-based cake, but without the calories. It has all the makings of a star: delicious, protein rich, quick, easy. The frosting is outstanding and super-low in calories. Best of all, it's an amazing treat that doesn't count as a cheat meal.

FOR THE CAKE

1 scoop casein protein powder, chocolate, vanilla, or cinnamon flavor

2 tablespoons milled flaxseed

½ cup water

⅓ cup egg whites

½ teaspoon vanilla extract

1 scoop whey isolate protein powder, chocolate

2 tablespoons unsweetened cocoa powder

2 tablespoons granulated stevia or Splenda

¼ teaspoon baking soda

Pinch ground cinnamon

FOR THE FROSTING

6 tablespoons Cool Whip Lite

3 tablespoons defatted peanut flour

3 tablespoons granulated stevia

5 drops vanilla extract

Nonfat Greek yogurt, as desired, to give it a cream cheese frosting taste (optional)

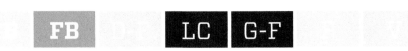

FB   **LC**   **G-F**

PER SERVING

Calories **124** Carbohydrates **8.2g** Fat **3.7g** Protein **17.1g**

¼ cake

TO MAKE THE CAKE

1 In a large mug, mix the casein, flaxseed, and water, and set aside to thicken for about 1 minute.

2 Add the egg whites, vanilla, whey, cocoa powder, stevia, baking soda, and cinnamon, and mix well.

3 Microwave in the mug for 2 to 3 minutes, depending on the depth of the cup. Keep an eye on it to prevent burning or drying out.

4 Cool completely, about 15 minutes, and then flip the cake over onto a plate.

TO MAKE THE FROSTING

1 In a small bowl mix the Cool Whip Lite, flour, stevia, vanilla, and yogurt (if using) until smooth.

2 Spread the frosting onto the cake, cut into four even pieces, and serve.

Time-saving tip: Spreading some plain peanut butter on top is a lower-fuss option that can be just as delicious. This option will change the overall calories and nutritional values.

Cooking tip: Ensure the cake has cooled completely before frosting. If it is still warm, the frosting will melt and slide off.

Ingredient tips: Not all protein powders are created equal. Choose wisely to ensure the best texture and flavor.

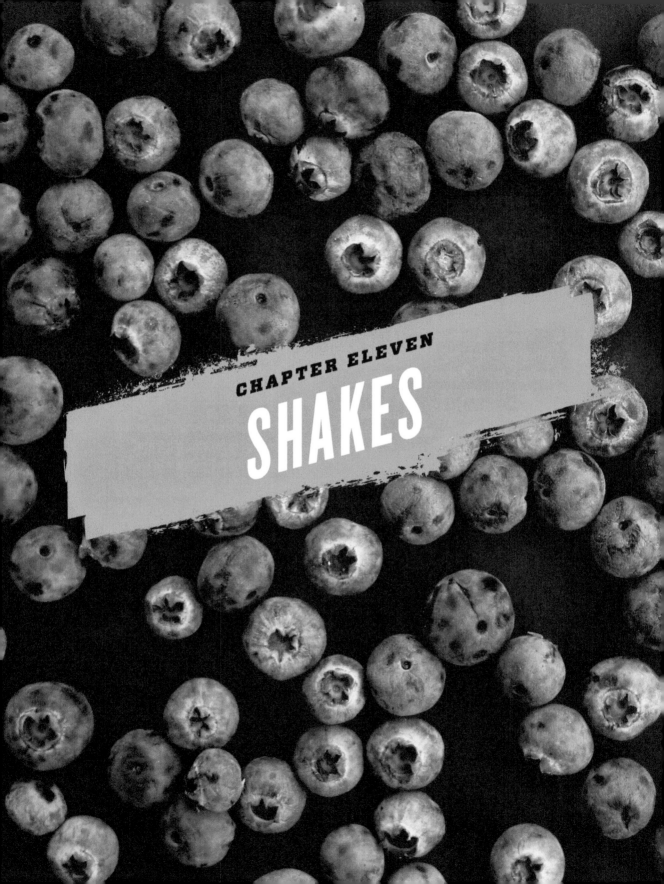

CHAPTER ELEVEN

SHAKES

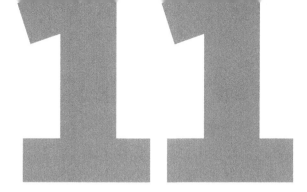

Shakes are convenient. Mix them up, drink them down, and you are on your way. Some of these recipes, however, taste so good you'll want to slowly sip and savor every last drop. From berries to beets, oatmeal to oranges, and chia to chocolate, your simple blender can create an impressive number of uniquely nutritious and delicious liquid meals.

If you have trouble getting all your vegetables in, smoothies are a great way to hide them in a handful of fruit. You can make a protein shake that tastes like a dessert from an ice cream parlor without any of the naughty nutrients. Each of the recipes in this chapter will give you a protein-packed way to blend up an amazing snack. Easy to digest, the nutrients will hit you fast, making them ideal for a pre- or post-workout meal. Don't forget, just because you don't have to chew it, doesn't mean it's not a meal. Remember to work these drinks into your meal plan.

MB Muscle Building **FB** Fat Burning **D-F** Dairy-Free **LC** Low Carb **G-F** Gluten-Free **P** Paleo **V** Vegan

CINNAMON AND SUGAR SHAKE

SERVES 1 / PREP TIME: 3 MINUTES

As creamy as a milkshake and as yummy as a cinnamon roll, this shake is full of protein and boosted with omega-3 fatty acids from flax seeds and pecans.

1 scoop casein protein powder, vanilla
   or cinnamon flavor
1 tablespoon milled flaxseed
¼ teaspoon ground cinnamon
¼ teaspoon vanilla extract
1 cup water
1 handful ice

1 In a blender, blend the protein powder, flaxseed, cinnamon, vanilla, water, and ice until smooth.

2 Pour into a glass and enjoy.

Ingredient tip: Use rice, casein, or other protein types with similar calorie composition, but it may change the texture and flavor.

FB   LC   G-F

PER SERVING

Calories **160** Carbohydrates **9g** Fat **2.2g** Protein **26.5g**

BANANA-NUT MUFFIN SHAKE

SERVES 1 / PREP TIME: 3 MINUTES

Ideal for pre-workout

Sweet and nutty, this filling shake has all the protein, carbs, and fat you need to get ready for a great workout.

10 raw unsalted almonds

1 cup unsweetened vanilla almond milk

½ banana

¼ cup whole rolled oatmeal

1 scoop whey isolate protein, vanilla
  or cinnamon flavor

1 handful ice

1 In a blender, blend the almonds, almond milk, banana, oatmeal, whey protein, and ice until smooth.

2 Pour into a glass and enjoy.

Ingredient tip: Use rice, casein, or other protein types with similar calorie composition, but it may change the texture and flavor.

MB   **G-F**

PER SERVING

Calories **312** Carbohydrates **28g** Fat **9g** Protein **30g**

WILD BERRY SMOOTHIE

SERVES 1 / PREP TIME: 3 MINUTES

Low in calories but high in protein, this shake makes a great snack and is full of antioxidant-filled berries.

1 scoop whey isolate protein powder, vanilla flavor

1½ cups water

½ cup nonfat Greek yogurt

¼ cup blueberries, fresh or frozen

¼ cup raspberries, fresh or frozen

¼ cup strawberries, fresh or frozen

2 tablespoons granulated stevia

1 handful ice (if using fresh berries)

1 In a blender, blend the protein powder, water, yogurt, berries, stevia, and ice (if using) until smooth.

2 Pour into a glass and enjoy.

Ingredient tip: *Use rice, casein, or other protein types with similar calorie composition, but it may change the texture and flavor.*

FB   G-F

PER SERVING

Calories **216** Carbohydrates **17g** Fat **1g** Protein **37g**

PROTEIN PUMPKIN-SPICE LATTE

SERVES 1 / PREP TIME: 3 MINUTES

Ideal for pre-workout

Why pay the barista $6 when you can make a protein-packed pumpkin spice latte at home? The coffee can give you a nice pick-me-up pre-workout boost—or any other time of day for that matter.

1 cup coffee, room temperature

1 scoop casein, vanilla flavor

1 tablespoon granulated stevia

¼ teaspoon ground cinnamon

⅛ teaspoon ground nutmeg

¼ teaspoon pumpkin flavor extract

1 handful ice

1 In a blender, blend the coffee, casein, stevia, cinnamon, nutmeg, pumpkin extract, and ice until smooth.

2 Pour into a glass and enjoy.

Cooking tip: *If you prefer your latte over ice instead of blended, combine all the ingredients in a shaker cup or blender EXCEPT the ice. Shake or blend until completely mixed, then pour the mixture over ice.*

Ingredient tips: *Flavor extracts can be found in your local grocery store's spice aisle.*

Use whey, rice, or other protein types with similar calorie composition, but it may change the texture and flavor.

FB **G-F** **V**

PER SERVING

Calories **120** Carbohydrates **4g** Fat **0g** Protein **24g**

PROTEIN PIÑA COLADA

SERVES 1 / PREP TIME: 3 MINUTES

Ideal for post-workout

It might be green, but the flavor is all piña colada. The pineapple masks the taste of the spinach and blends with the creamy coconut to deliver lots of healthy fats, protein, vitamins, and minerals.

1 scoop casein protein powder, vanilla flavor

1 cup tightly packed baby spinach

1 cup pineapple chunks, fresh or frozen

1 cup water

¼ cup reduced-fat unsweetened coconut milk

2 tablespoons granulated stevia (optional)

1 handful ice (if using fresh pineapple)

1 In a blender, blend the casein, spinach, pineapple, water, coconut milk, stevia, and ice (if using) until smooth.

2 Pour into a glass and enjoy.

Ingredient tips: *The coconut milk you want to purchase can be found at your local grocery store in the ethnic food aisle. It comes in a can. It is not the same coconut milk in cartons you would find next to the almond and soy milk.*

Use whey, rice, or other protein types with similar calorie composition, but it may change the texture and flavor.

MB   **G-F**

PER SERVING

Calories **253** Carbohydrates **29g** Fat **10g** Protein **27g**

PROTEIN HORCHATA

SERVES 1 / PREP TIME: 3 MINUTES

This nod to the classic Hispanic drink—with a protein twist—has all the great flavor without any of the added sugar.

1½ cups unsweetened almond milk

1 scoop whey protein isolate, vanilla flavor

1 to 2 tablespoons granulated stevia

½ teaspoon ground cinnamon

¼ teaspoon vanilla extract

1 In a shaker cup or blender, shake or blend the almond milk, protein powder, stevia, cinnamon, and vanilla until smooth.

2 Pour into a glass and enjoy.

Cooking tip: *If prefer your drink colder, add ice to the shaker after you have blended the drink. Shake for 20 seconds, and then pour into a glass. You could also serve over ice or blend with ice.*

Ingredient tip: *Use casein, rice, or other protein types with similar calorie composition, but it may change the texture and flavor.*

FB   **LC** **G-F**

PER SERVING

Calories **150** Carbohydrates **5g** Fat **3g** Protein **25g**

PEACHES 'N' CREAM SHAKE

SERVES 1 / PREP TIME: 3 MINUTES

Sweet ripe peaches with rich and creamy casein make this shake a delicious way to cool down after a workout.

1 scoop casein protein powder,
  vanilla flavor
1 cup (1 to 2) peaches, fresh or frozen
1½ cups water
Granulated stevia, as desired
1 handful ice (if using fresh peaches)

1 In a blender, blend the casein, peaches, water, stevia, and ice (if using) until smooth.

2 Pour into a glass and enjoy.

Ingredient tips: *Fresh, ripe peaches will taste much better than frozen.*

Use whey, rice, or other protein types with similar calorie composition, but it may change the texture and flavor.

FB **LC** **G-F**

PER SERVING

Calories **180** Carbohydrates **19g** Fat **2g** Protein **25g**

THE BIG GREEN SMOOTHIE

SERVES 1 / PREP TIME: 3 MINUTES

Ideal for post-workout

Fruits, veggies, and protein feed your muscles post-workout. With the refreshing blend of orange, apple, and ginger, you won't even taste the spinach.

2 cups baby spinach

1 cup water

1 cup egg whites

1 large orange, peeled and sectioned

1 large Fuji apple

½ teaspoon fresh ginger

1 handful ice

1 In a blender, blend the spinach, water, egg whites, orange, apple, ginger, and ice until smooth.

2 Pour into a glass and enjoy.

MB **G-F** **P**

PER SERVING

Calories **289** Carbohydrates **44g** Fat **1g** Protein **29g**

STRAWBERRY CHEESECAKE SHAKE

SERVES 1 / PREP TIME: 3 MINUTES

Creamy and delicious, this shake brims with naturally sweet strawberry flavor perfectly balanced with the smooth tang of Greek yogurt.

1 scoop casein protein powder, vanilla or strawberry flavor

8 frozen strawberries

1½ cups water

⅓ cup nonfat Greek yogurt

2 tablespoons granulated stevia

1 In a blender, blend the casein, strawberries, water, yogurt, and stevia until smooth.

2 Pour into a glass and enjoy.

Ingredient tip: *Use whey, rice, or other protein types with similar calorie composition, but it may change the texture and flavor.*

FB **G-F**

PER SERVING

Calories **212** Carbohydrates **19g** Fat **2g** Protein **33g**

PEANUT BUTTER–NUTELLA SHAKE

SERVES 1 / PREP TIME: 3 MINUTES

If you dream of digging into a jar of peanut butter and following it with a big spoonful of Nutella, this is the shake for you! All the chocolate, hazelnut, and peanut butter goodness, without any of the fat or sugar and with a healthy scoop of protein, elevates this to the pantheon of guilt-free pleasures.

1¼ cups water

1 scoop whey protein isolate, chocolate flavor

¼ cup defatted peanut butter

2 tablespoons granulated stevia

½ teaspoon hazelnut extract

1 In a blender, blend the water, protein powder, peanut butter, stevia, and hazelnut extract until smooth.

2 Pour into a glass and enjoy.

Ingredient tips: Flavor extracts can be found in your local grocery store's spice aisle.

Use rice, casein, or other protein types with similar calorie composition, but it may change the texture and flavor.

FB   LC   G-F

PER SERVING

Calories **154** Carbohydrates **6g** Fat **0g** Protein **33g**

BLUEBERRIES AND BEETS SMOOTHIE

SERVES 1 / PREP TIME: 3 MINUTES

Ideal for pre-workout

This shake has all you need—beets to give your muscles a big nitric oxide boost of power and endurance; protein, carbs, and fats to fuel your muscles to prepare for an intense workout.

1 cup blueberries, fresh or frozen

½ cup canned beets with liquids

1 scoop whey protein isolate, chocolate flavor

1 tablespoon chia seeds

2 tablespoons honey

1 handful ice (if using fresh blueberries)

1 In a blender, blend the blueberries, beets, protein powder, chia seeds, honey, and ice (if using) until smooth.

2 Pour into a glass and enjoy.

Ingredient tips: *Fresh beets work great as well.*

Use whey, casein, or other protein types with similar calorie composition, but it may change the texture and flavor.

MB   G-F

PER SERVING

Calories **349** Carbohydrates **39g** Fat **5g** Protein **27g**

NUTS ABOUT HONEY SHAKE

SERVES 1 / PREP TIME: 3 MINUTES

Ideal for pre-workout

Loaded with all you need for a great workout, this shake is as creamy as a milkshake, and just as yummy. Better yet, the fats, protein, and carbs are all in harmonious balance.

10 raw unsalted cashews

1 scoop casein protein, vanilla or cinnamon flavor

¼ cup whole rolled oats

1 tablespoon honey

¼ teaspoon ground cinnamon

1 cup water

1 handful of ice

1 In a blender, blend the cashews, casein, oats, honey, cinnamon, water, and ice until smooth.

2 Pour into a glass and enjoy.

Ingredient tip: *Use whey, rice, or other protein types with similar calorie composition, but it may change the texture and flavor.*

MB   **G-F**

PER SERVING

Calories **349** Carbohydrates **39g** Fat **10g** Protein **27g**

ROOT BEER FLOAT SHAKE

SERVES 1 / PREP TIME: 3 MINUTES

Cold, creamy, and full of the root beer flavor, enjoy this old-fashioned dessert without any worry of added sugar or empty calories.

1 cup unsweetened almond milk

1 scoop casein protein powder, vanilla flavor

10 raw unsalted cashews

1 Medjool date, pitted

½ teaspoon root beer extract, or more if desired

1 handful ice

1 In a blender, blend the almond milk, casein, cashews, date, root beer extract, and ice until smooth.

2 Pour into a glass and enjoy.

Ingredient tips: Flavor extracts can be found in your local grocery store's spice aisle.

Use whey, rice, or other protein types with similar calorie composition, but it may change the texture and flavor.

FB   **G-F**

PER SERVING

Calories **292** Carbohydrates **17g** Fat **13g** Protein **30g**

BLUEBERRY MUFFIN SHAKE

SERVES 1 / PREP TIME: 3 MINUTES

Ideal for pre-workout

This shake has fresh antioxidant-rich blueberries blended up with creamy casein. It's full of fiber, healthy fats, oats, and plenty of protein to fuel your mornings.

½ cup blueberries, fresh or frozen

1 scoop casein protein powder, vanilla flavor

¼ cup whole rolled oats

1 tablespoon milled flaxseed

1 tablespoon psyllium husk

1 tablespoon granulated stevia

1½ cups water

1 handful ice (if using fresh blueberries)

1 In a blender, blend the blueberries, casein, oats, flaxseed, psyllium, stevia, water, and ice (if using) until smooth.

2 Pour into a glass and serve.

MB

G-F

PER SERVING

Calories **278** Carbohydrates **30g** Fat **6g** Protein **30g**

ORANGE CREAMSICLE SHAKE

SERVES 1 / PREP TIME: 3 MINUTES

As refreshing as an orange creamsicle on a hot summer day, this shake has a nice blend of whey, casein, and coconut milk that creates a thick, creamy texture as good as ice cream itself.

½ scoop whey protein isolate, vanilla flavor

½ scoop casein protein, vanilla flavor

⅔ cup orange juice

¼ cup light coconut milk

1 to 2 tablespoons granulated stevia

1 handful ice

1 In a blender, blend the protein powder, casein, orange juice, coconut milk, stevia, and ice until smooth.

2 Pour into a glass and enjoy.

FB   G-F

PER SERVING

Calories **230** Carbohydrates **20g** Fat **5g** Protein **26g**

RASPBERRY-ORANGE SHAKE

SERVES 1 / PREP TIME: 3 MINUTES

Loaded with citrus, raspberry ketones, and lean egg white protein, this delicious smoothie will turn up your metabolism and help break down fat cells.

1 cup pasteurized egg whites

1 cup raspberries, fresh or frozen

¼ cup orange juice

1 tablespoon granulated stevia

1 handful ice (if using fresh raspberries)

1 In a blender, blend the egg whites, raspberries, orange juice, stevia, and ice (if using) until smooth.

2 Pour into a glass and serve.

Ingredient tip: For extra fiber, use a few slices of real orange instead of orange juice.

FB   G-F   V

PER SERVING

Calories **218** Carbohydrates **23g** Fat **1g** Protein **28g**

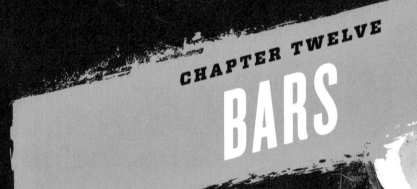

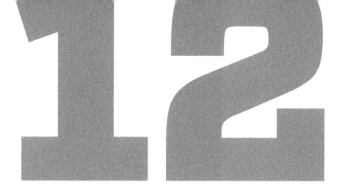

Easily tossed in your pocket, purse, or gym bag for a quick bite anywhere the day takes you, bars are a convenient way to get a healthy boost on the go. Making your own bars at home guarantees they're made from the best ingredients and eliminates all the chemical dyes and preservatives that store-bought bars use to lengthen shelf life. Dollar for dollar, homemade bars can also save you quite a few bucks in the long run.

To get the most from your bars, make sure you work them appropriately into your overall calories and time them properly for your nutritional needs. Bars with a higher amount of carbohydrates are best to refuel after a hard workout, while bars that are high in protein and relatively low in carbohydrates are a more suitable snack for other times of the day. Each recipe in this chapter is inspired by favorite desserts and name brand bars.

MB Muscle Building **FB** Fat Burning **D-F** Dairy-Free **LC** Low Carb **G-F** Gluten-Free **P** Paleo **V** Vegan

SNICKERDOODLE BARS

MAKES 4 BARS / PREP TIME: 10 MINUTES, PLUS 30 MINUTES TO CHILL

Based on the old-fashioned cookie recipe, this bar is sweet, cinnamony, and oh-so-delicious. It's a low-calorie, high-fiber protein snack you can enjoy any time of the day.

2 scoops whey protein isolate powder, vanilla flavor

½ cup raw unsalted cashews

½ cup almond flour

2 teaspoons ground cinnamon

¼ cup IMO syrup

Ingredient tips: IMO stands for Isomalto-oligosaccharide. It is a high-fiber, low-calorie sweetener commonly used in the most popular protein bars available in stores. IMO can be made from several forms of vegetable starches and is available at popular online retailers.

Not all protein powder is created equal. Choose wisely. The taste and texture will make a big difference in the final product.

Cooking tip: Multiply this recipe to create your desired number of bars.

1 In a food processor or blender, process the whey protein, cashews, almond flour, and cinnamon until a flour consistency is reached. Transfer to a large bowl.

2 Pour the IMO syrup over the dry ingredients. Using a spoon, mix until a thick, sticky batter forms and the batter is well mixed.

3 Using your hands, form the batter into 4 evenly sized bars and place them in individual resealable bags. Refrigerate for at least 30 minutes, until firm.

4 Store for up to 1 week in the refrigerator or 1 month in the freezer.

FB   **LC**   **G-F**

PER SERVING

Calories **195** Carbohydrates **8.5g** Fat **11g** Protein **16.8g**

1 bar

TROPICAL ISLAND CRUNCH BARS

MAKES 10 BARS / PREP TIME: 10 MINUTES /
COOK TIME: 15 MINUTES / TOTAL TIME: 40 MINUTES

Ideal for post-workout

Carbs from the pineapple, oats, and rice replenish you post-workout, while the healthy fats and protein will hold you over until your next meal.

Extra-virgin olive oil spray
1 cup whole rolled oats
1 cup crisp rice cereal
½ cup raw unsalted almonds, slivered
¼ cup macadamia nuts, chopped
¼ cup unsweetened shredded coconut
¼ cup crystallized pineapple, chopped
2 tablespoons coconut oil
¼ cup honey or agave
¼ cup unsweetened vanilla almond milk
2 scoops whey isolate protein powder, vanilla flavor

Ingredient tip: Not all protein powder is created equal. Choose wisely. The taste and texture will make a big difference in the final product.

1 Preheat the oven to 325°F.

2 Lightly coat a baking sheet with olive oil spray.

3 In a large bowl, mix the oats, crisp rice cereal, almonds, macadamia nuts, coconut, and pineapple. Set aside.

4 In a small saucepan over medium-low heat, melt the coconut oil. Whisk in the honey and almond milk until smooth. Whisk in the protein powder until smooth.

5 Stir the protein mixture into the oat and rice cereal mixture.

6 Using wet hands, press the mixture firmly into 10 evenly sized bars, about 4 by 2 inches each, and place them on the prepared sheet.

7 Bake for 15 minutes, until the bars start to turn golden.

8 Let cool for 15 minutes, and then transfer to a storage container or resealable bags. Store in the refrigerator for up to 1 week or the freezer for up to 1 month.

MB

G-F

PER SERVING

Calories **300** Carbohydrates **24.4g** Fat **18.8g** Protein **11.5g**

1 bar

OATMEAL COOKIE BARS

**MAKES 10 BARS / PREP TIME: 10 MINUTES /
COOK TIME: 15 MINUTES / TOTAL TIME: 40 MINUTES**

Ideal for pre-workout

These home-baked bars that taste like fresh oatmeal cookies are a well-balanced mix of carbs, fat, and protein. It's the perfect pre-workout bar, giving you just enough energy to power through a workout without weighing you down.

Extra-virgin olive oil spray

2 cups whole rolled oats

½ cup raw unsalted walnuts, chopped

¼ cup dried cranberries or raisins

1 teaspoon ground cinnamon

2 tablespoons coconut oil

2 tablespoons maple syrup

2 tablespoons honey

¼ cup unsweetened vanilla
  almond milk

2 scoops whey protein isolate powder,
  cinnamon or vanilla flavor

1 Preheat the oven to 325°F.

2 Lightly coat a baking sheet with olive oil spray.

3 In a large bowl, mix the oats, walnuts, cranberries, and cinnamon. Set aside.

4 In a small saucepan over medium-low heat, heat the coconut oil. Whisk in the maple syrup, honey, and almond milk until smooth. Whisk in the protein powder until smooth.

MB   **G-F**

PER SERVING   Calories **143** Carbohydrates **14.3g** Fat **7.3g** Protein **6.9g**   1 bar

5 Add the protein mixture to the oat mixture, and stir well. Transfer to the prepared baking sheet. Using wet hands, press the mixture firmly into 10 evenly sized bars. Bars can be rectangular, or you can form balls and press them flat like a cookie.

6 Bake for 12 to 15 minutes, until the bars start to turn golden.

7 Let cool for 10 minutes, and then transfer to a storage container or resealable bags. Store in the refrigerator for up to 1 week or in the freezer for up to 1 month.

Ingredient tip: *Not all protein powder is created equal. Choose wisely. The taste and texture will make a big difference in the final product.*

PEANUT BUTTER AND MAPLE BALLS

MAKES 10 BALLS / PREP TIME: 10 MINUTES, PLUS 10 MINUTES TO CHILL

Ideal for post-workout

These no-bake snack balls make the perfect snack for a quick burst of energy post-workout. Peanut butter and maple syrup are a yummy combination, and these balls are a great way to reacquaint the two.

1½ cups oat flour

½ cup defatted peanut flour

½ cup crisp rice cereal

½ teaspoon salt, or as desired

½ cup natural peanut butter or other nut butter

½ cup maple syrup

1 teaspoon vanilla extract

Ingredient tips: If you don't have oat flour on hand, you can make your own by blending whole oats in a food processor or blender.

A natural peanut butter has only one ingredient—dry-roasted peanuts. It could also have salt for taste. Avoid peanut butters with any other ingredients.

Cooking tip: If you prefer a different shape, press the batter into a baking dish and cut into square bars.

1 In a large bowl, mix the oat flour, peanut flour, crisp rice cereal, and salt.

2 Add the peanut butter, maple syrup, and vanilla, and stir until it resembles a cookie dough.

3 Using your hands, roll the batter into 10 evenly sized balls. Freeze for 5 to 10 minutes.

4 Remove from the freezer, and transfer to resealable bags or a storage container. Store in the refrigerator for 1 week or in the freezer for up to 1 month.

MB **G-F** **V**

PER SERVING

Calories **195** Carbohydrates **26.2g** Fat **7.8g** Protein **8g**

1 ball

ALMOND BUTTER AND HONEY CRISPS

MAKES 10 BARS / PREP TIME: 10 MINUTES, PLUS 10 MINUTES TO CHILL

Ideal for post-workout

Sweet honey and almond butter blend to make the perfect bar. The rice gives it a crispy texture and pumps up the batter volume. Psyllium husk punches up the fiber content, helping you feel full longer.

1 cup oat flour

¼ cup psyllium husk

2 scoops whey protein isolate powder, vanilla or cinnamon flavor

2 cups crisp rice cereal

¾ cup natural almond butter or other nut butter

¼ cup honey

½ teaspoon ground cinnamon (optional)

Ingredient tips: *If you don't have oat flour on hand, you can make your own by grinding whole oats in a food processor or blender.*

A natural almond butter has only one ingredient: dry-roasted almonds. It could also have salt for taste. Avoid almond butters with any other ingredients.

1 Line a baking sheet with parchment paper or a silicone baking sheet.

2 In a large bowl, mix the oat flour, psyllium husk, protein powder, and crisp rice cereal.

3 Add the almond butter and honey. Mix until crumbly clumps form.

4 Using your hands, gather the batter into a ball. Transfer to the prepared baking sheet. Using your hands to press or a rolling pin, make a rectangle. Freeze for 5 to 10 minutes, or if it will not fit in the freezer, refrigerate for 15 to 20 minutes.

5 Cut into 10 evenly sized bars, and transfer to resealable bags or a storage container. Store in the refrigerator for 1 week or in the freezer for up to 1 month.

Cooking tip: *If you prefer a different shape, roll the dough into balls or hand-shape them into individual bars.*

MB   **G-F**   **V**

PER SERVING

Calories **250** Carbohydrates **25.6g** Fat **11.8g** Protein **11.7g**

1 bar

CHEWY GOOEY FUDGE BARS

MAKES 10 BARS / PREP TIME: 10 MINUTES

Ideal for post-workout

As gooey and rich as your favorite fudge, these bars taste so good it's hard to believe they are good for you. Enjoy one after your workout with your favorite protein.

1 cup oat flour

1 scoop whey isolate protein powder, chocolate flavor

¼ cup natural unsweetened cocoa powder

14 Medjool dates, pitted

¾ cup raw unsalted walnuts, halved or chopped, divided

1 teaspoon vanilla extract

½ teaspoon salt

½ teaspoon ground cinnamon

¼ cup chocolate chips

Ingredient tips: If you don't have oat flour on hand, you can make your own by grinding whole oats in a food processor or blender.

The best dates to get are Medjool dates. Try to find the moistest ones you can.

1 Line a baking sheet with parchment paper.

2 In a food processor or blender, process the oat flour, protein powder, and cocoa powder until well mixed.

3 Add the dates, ½ cup of walnuts, and the vanilla, salt, and cinnamon. Process until a thick dough forms.

4 Transfer the dough to the prepared baking sheet. Using your hands, knead in the remaining ¼ cup of walnuts and the chocolate chips, and then shape the dough into a square. A larger square will result in thinner bars.

5 Gently cut into 10 evenly sized bars, and transfer to resealable bags or an airtight storage container. Store for up to 1 week in the refrigerator or 1 month in the freezer.

MB **G-F** **V**

PER SERVING

Calories **166** Carbohydrates **27.7g** Fat **6.1g** Protein **4.9g**

1 bar

CHEWY APPLE TURNOVER BARS

MAKES 8 BARS / PREP TIME: 5 MINUTES, PLUS 30 MINUTES TO CHILL

Ideal for post-workout

These no-bake bars pair delicious apple cinnamon flavors with nutritious and filling nutty goodness. Enjoy them post-workout paired with your favorite protein shake.

½ cup raw unsalted walnuts
½ cup raw unsalted pecans
1 teaspoon ground cinnamon
¼ teaspoon salt, or as desired
14 Medjool dates, pitted
¾ cup dried apple

1 Line a baking sheet with plastic wrap or parchment paper.

2 In a food processor or blender, pulse the walnuts, pecans, cinnamon, and salt a few times, until the nuts are chopped into large pieces.

3 Add the dates and apple, a few at time, pulsing between additions. Once all the dates and apple have been added, process until you have a thick mixture that sticks together.

4 Spoon the mixture onto the prepared baking sheet, and using your hands, form an 8-inch square. Cover with a second piece of plastic wrap or parchment paper. (For presentation, if you prefer, you can use a roller to smooth out the mixture.)

5 Refrigerate for 30 minutes or more.

6 Cut into 8 bars, each about 4 by 2 inches. Wrap the bars in plastic wrap or transfer to individual resealable bags so they don't stick together. Store in the refrigerator for up to a few weeks.

Ingredient tips: *Get the gooiest, most moist dates you can find.*

The dried apple should be chewy, not dry chips.

MB   **G-F** **P** **V**

PER SERVING

Calories **226** Carbohydrates **38g** Fat **9,2g** Protein **3g**

1 bar

CHOCOLATE–PEANUT BUTTER CRISPY BARS

MAKES 10 BARS / PREP TIME: 3 MINUTES

Ideal for post-workout

This no-bake bar is chocolaty and full of texture, and it leaves you with that yummy, gooey, peanut butter flavor we all crave. Treat yourself with a little chocolate drizzle on top. After a hard workout, you deserve it.

1 cup oat flour

½ cup whole rolled oats

3 scoops whey isolate protein powder, chocolate flavor

½ cup crisp rice cereal

¼ cup honey

⅓ cup peanut butter or other nut butter

1 teaspoon vanilla extract

6 tablespoons water, divided

2 tablespoons chocolate chips

Ingredient tips: If you don't have oat flour on hand, you can make your own by blending whole oats in a food processor or blender.

A natural peanut butter has only one ingredient—dry-roasted peanuts. It could also have salt for taste. Avoid any peanut butters with anything else in them.

MB　**G-F**

PER SERVING

Calories **186** Carbohydrates **22.8g** Fat **6.1g** Protein **12.2g**

1 bar

1 Line a baking sheet with parchment paper.

2 In a large bowl, mix the oat flour, rolled oats, protein powder, and crisp rice cereal. Set aside.

3 In a small saucepan over medium-low heat, stir the honey, peanut butter, and vanilla until smooth.

4 Stir the peanut butter mixture into the oat mixture.

5 Add the water 1 tablespoon at a time, stirring after each addition, until a thick batter forms. You may not need all the water.

6 Transfer the dough to the prepared baking sheet. Using your hands, shape the dough into a square. A larger square will result in thinner bars.

7 In a small microwavable bowl, melt the chocolate chips in the microwave on high for 1 minute. Using a spoon, drizzle the melted chocolate over the dough, or spread it out over all.

8 Refrigerate for 15 minutes.

9 Cut into 10 evenly sized squares, and transfer to resealable bags or a storage container. Store for up to 1 week in the refrigerator or 1 month in the freezer.

CHEWY SWEET CINNAMON BARS

MAKES 8 BARS / PREP TIME: 5 MINUTES, PLUS 30 MINUTES TO CHILL

Ideal for post-workout

This bar is sweet and smooth, with a touch of cinnamon. Dates, cashews, and almonds create a rich and creamy flavor that will satisfy your sweet tooth. Pair one with your favorite proteins for a terrific post-workout snack.

½ **cup raw unsalted almonds**
½ **cup raw unsalted cashews**
1 **tablespoon ground cinnamon**
¼ **teaspoon salt, or less as desired**
1 **teaspoon vanilla extract**
14 **Medjool dates, pitted**

1 Line a baking sheet with plastic wrap or parchment paper.

2 In a food processor or blender, pulse the almonds, cashews, cinnamon, salt, and vanilla a few times, until the nuts are chopped into large pieces.

3 Add the dates a few at a time, processing after each addition. Once all the dates have been added, process until you have a thick mixture that sticks together.

4 Spoon the mixture onto the prepared baking sheet, and using your hands, form an 8-inch square. Cover with a second piece of plastic wrap or parchment paper. (For presentation, if you prefer, you can use a roller to smooth out the mixture.)

5 Refrigerate for 30 minutes or more.

6 Cut into 8 evenly sized bars, each about 4 by 2 inches. Wrap the bars in plastic wrap or transfer to individual resealable bags so they don't stick together. Store the bars in the refrigerator for up to a few weeks.

Ingredient tip: *Get the gooiest, most moist dates you can find.*

MB **G-F** **P** **V**

PER SERVING

Calories **208** Carbohydrates **35g** Fat **7.8g** Protein **3.8g**

1 bar

CHEWY COCONUT BARS

MAKES 8 BARS / PREP TIME: 5 MINUTES, PLUS 30 MINUTES TO CHILL

Ideal for post-workout

Naturally sweet, silky coconut is paired with rich and chewy dates in this delectable bar. Healthy fats and fiber satisfy your hunger, while the sweet dates pick up your energy after a long workout. Pair one with your favorite protein for the perfect post-workout snack.

½ **cup raw unsalted almonds**
½ **cup raw unsalted cashews**
½ **cup unsweetened shredded coconut**
¼ **teaspoon vanilla extract**
14 Medjool dates, pitted

1 Line a baking sheet with plastic wrap or parchment paper.

2 In a food processor or blender, pulse the almonds, cashews, and shredded coconut a few times, until the nuts are chopped into large pieces.

3 With the food processor running, add the vanilla extract and dates. Process until you have a thick mixture that sticks together.

4 Spoon the mixture onto the prepared baking sheet, and using your hands, form the mixture into an 8-inch square. Cover with a second piece of plastic wrap or parchment paper. (For presentation, if you prefer, you can use a roller to smooth out the mixture.)

5 Refrigerate for 30 minutes or more.

6 Cut into 8 bars, each about 4 by 2 inches. Wrap the bars in plastic wrap or transfer to individual resealable bags so they don't stick together. Store the bars in the refrigerator for up to a few weeks, or in the freezer for a few months.

Ingredient tip: *Get the gooiest, most moist dates you can find.*

MB   **G-F**   **P**   **V**

PER SERVING

Calories **225** Carbohydrates **36.1g** Fat **9.5g** Protein **4.1g**

1 bar

DARK CHOCOLATE–RASPBERRY TRUFFLE BARS

**MAKES 5 TRUFFLES / PREP TIME: 5 MINUTES /
COOK TIME: 2 MINUTES, PLUS 30 MINUTES TO CHILL**

With a soft raspberry-filled center surrounded by a dark chocolate shell, this decadent treat has an even balance of all your macronutrients and will leave you feeling pampered.

1 scoop whey isolate protein powder, vanilla or berry flavor

½ cup almond flour, divided

2 tablespoons coconut flour

1 tablespoon granulated stevia

½ cup raspberries, fresh or frozen

1½ teaspoons vanilla extract

2 tablespoons dark chocolate chips

Ingredient tips: For a softer texture in the truffle, you could replace the coconut flour with more almond flour.

If you are using frozen raspberries, heat them in the microwave for 1 minute prior to adding them to the batter.

If you prefer milk chocolate instead, it will change the nutritional values.

MB **G-F**

PER SERVING

Calories **131** Carbohydrates **9.2g** Fat **8g** Protein **8.2g**

1 truffle

1 Line a baking sheet with parchment paper or a silicone baking mat.

2 In a medium bowl, stir the protein powder and 6 tablespoons of almond flour together with the coconut flour and stevia.

3 Add the raspberries and vanilla extract. Using a fork, stir until a thick, sticky dough forms.

4 Lightly dust the prepared baking sheet with the remaining 2 tablespoons of almond flour. Transfer the dough to the baking sheet, and roll it around so that it is very lightly coated with just enough almond flour to make it no longer sticky. Using your hands, shape it into a long, narrow rectangle, about 10 by 2 inches. Using a butter knife, cut the dough into 5 pieces, each 2 by 2 inches.

5 In a small microwavable bowl, melt the chocolate in the microwave for 1 to 2 minutes. Dip each square of the dough into the chocolate to lightly coat, and place back on the baking sheet.

6 Refrigerate for 30 minutes, until the chocolate hardens.

7 Transfer to a storage container or resealable bags, and store in the refrigerator for up to 1 week.

BANANA BREAD BARS

MAKES 8 BARS / PREP TIME: 10 MINUTES, PLUS 15 MINUTES TO CHILL

Ideal for pre-workout

A delicious no-bake banana bread bar that is soft, fudgy, and healthy, too? Yes! This bar also delivers loads of energy for such a small pre-workout snack.

¼ cup (a little under 1 medium overripe) banana, mashed
½ cup almond flour
¼ cup cashew butter or other nut butter
2 scoops brown rice protein, vanilla flavor

Ingredient tips: *Place the overripe peeled banana in a medium bowl. Using a fork, mash until relatively smooth. Measure out ¼ cup.*

The scoop size of rice protein can vary. One scoop should have about 24 grams of protein.

1 Line a baking sheet with plastic wrap or parchment paper.

2 In a medium bowl, mix the banana and almond flour until well-incorporated but crumbly.

3 In a small saucepan over medium-low heat, stir the cashew butter and protein until melted and smooth. Stir into the banana mixture until well-incorporated and a thick batter forms.

4 Spoon the mixture onto the prepared baking sheet, and using your hands, form the mixture into an 8-inch square. Cover with a second piece of plastic wrap or parchment paper. (For presentation, if you prefer, you can use a roller to smooth out the mixture.)

5 Refrigerate for 15 minutes, until firm.

6 Cut into eight evenly sized squares, and transfer to storage containers or resealable bags. Store for up to 1 week in the refrigerator or 1 month in the freezer.

MB **LC** **G-F** **V**

PER SERVING

Calories **120** Carbohydrates **5.6g** Fat **7.7g** Protein **9.6g**

1 bar

LEMON BAR COOKIES

MAKES 4 COOKIES / PREP TIME: 15 MINUTES, PLUS 15 MINUTES TO CHILL

Ideal for batch cooking

So delicious they taste like the real deal, these cookies have that zesty zing that makes lemon bars hard to pass up. Loads of protein make this an excellent pre-workout snack.

2 scoops whey protein isolate powder, vanilla flavor

½ cup raw unsalted cashews

¼ cup almond flour

Zest of 1 large lemon, plus ¼ cup freshly squeezed lemon juice, divided

1 In a food processor or blender, process the whey protein, cashews, almond flour, and lemon zest until well-mixed. Transfer to a medium bowl.

2 Sir in the lemon juice gradually, mixing until a thick dough forms.

3 Using your hands, form the batter into four balls. Place them on a plate and flatten into cookies. Refrigerate for at least 15 minutes, until firm.

4 Transfer to a storage container or resealable bag, and store for up to 1 week in the refrigerator or 1 month in the freezer.

Ingredient tip: *Not all protein powder is created equal. Choose wisely. The taste and texture will make a big difference in the final product.*

FB　**G-F**

PER SERVING

Calories **195**　Carbohydrates **8.5g**　Fat **11g**　Protein **16.8g**

1 cookie

PEANUT BUTTER CUP BARS

MAKES 4 BARS / PREP TIME: 10 MINUTES, PLUS 30 MINUTES TO CHILL

Ideal for batch cooking

If you are on a quest to make a homemade protein bar that tastes just as good as your favorite store-bought brand, search no more. The secret ingredient is the high-fiber, low-calorie sweetener IMO. This is a great protein snack for any time of the day.

2 scoops whey protein isolate powder, chocolate flavor
½ cup defatted peanut flour
¼ cup almond flour
¼ cup IMO syrup
¼ cup unsweetened vanilla almond milk

Ingredient tips: IMO stands for Isomalto-oligosaccharide. It is a high-fiber, low-calorie sweetener commonly used in the most popular protein bars available in stores. IMO can be made from several forms of vegetable starches and is available at popular online retailers.

Not all protein powder is created equal. Choose wisely. The taste and texture will make a big difference in the final product.

1 In a medium bowl, mix the protein powder, peanut flour, and almond flour.

2 Pour the IMO syrup and almond milk over the dry ingredients. Using a spoon, mix until a thick, sticky batter forms.

3 Using wet hands, form the batter into four evenly sized bars and place them in individual resealable bags. Refrigerate for at least 30 minutes, until firm.

4 Store for up to 1 week in the refrigerator or 1 month in the freezer.

FB **LC** **G-F**

PER SERVING

Calories **130** Carbohydrates **10g** Fat **3.8g** Protein **18g**

1 bar

STRAWBERRY CHEESECAKE BARS

MAKES 4 BARS / PREP TIME: 10 MINUTES, PLUS 30 MINUTES TO CHILL

Ideal for batch cooking

Creamy vanilla and real strawberries give this dessert-quality treat protein-bar nutrition. IMO syrup makes it a great protein snack any time of the day.

2 scoops whey protein isolate powder, vanilla flavor
½ cup raw unsalted cashews
½ cup almond flour
½ cup dried strawberries, divided
¼ cup IMO syrup

Ingredient tips: *IMO stands for Isomalto-oligosaccharide. It is a high-fiber, low-calorie sweetener commonly used in the most popular protein bars available in stores. IMO can be made from several forms of vegetable starches and is available at popular online retailers.*

Not all protein powder is created equal. Choose wisely. The taste and texture will make a big difference in the final product.

1 In a food processor or blender, process the whey protein, cashews, almond flour, and ¼ cup of dried strawberries until a flour is reached. Transfer to a large bowl.

2 Pour the IMO syrup over the dry ingredients. Using a spoon, mix until a thick, sticky batter forms. Add the remaining ¼ cup of dried strawberries, and using your hands, knead until well mixed.

3 Using your hands, form the batter into four evenly sized bars and place them in individual resealable bags. Refrigerate for at least 30 minutes, until firm.

4 Store for up to 1 week in the refrigerator or 1 month in the freezer.

FB **LC** **G-F**

PER SERVING

Calories **205** Carbohydrates **8.5g** Fat **11g** Protein **16.8g**

1 bar

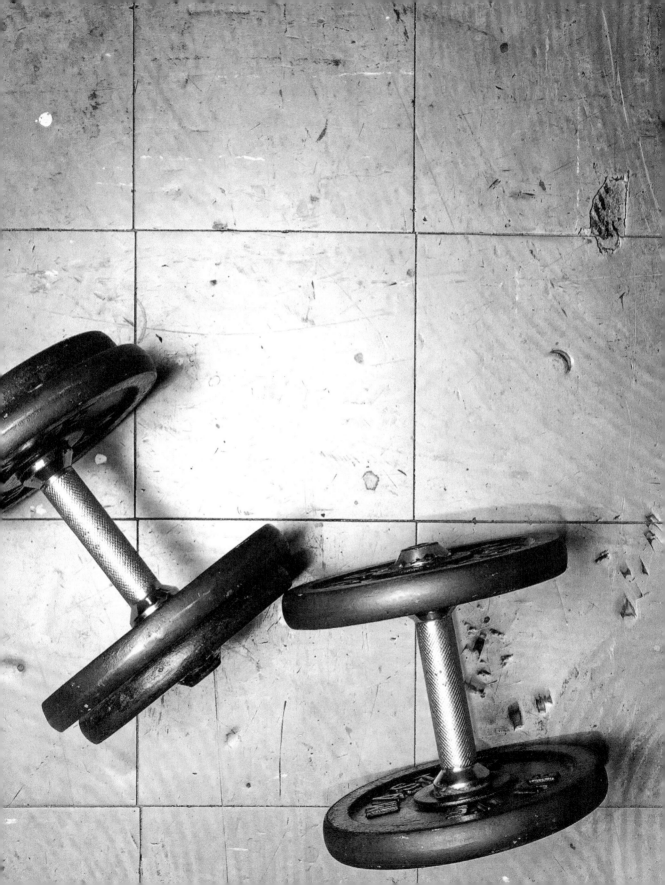

CONVERSIONS

VOLUME EQUIVALENTS (LIQUID)

US STANDARD	US STANDARD (OUNCES)	METRIC (APPROXIMATE)
2 tablespoons	1 fl. oz.	30 mL
¼ cup	2 fl. oz.	60 mL
½ cup	4 fl. oz.	120 mL
1 cup	8 fl. oz.	240 mL
1½ cups	12 fl. oz.	355 mL
2 cups or 1 pint	16 fl. oz.	475 mL
4 cups or 1 quart	32 fl. oz.	1 L
1 gallon	128 fl. oz.	4 L

VOLUME EQUIVALENTS (DRY)

US STANDARD	METRIC (APPROXIMATE)
⅛ teaspoon	0.5 mL
¼ teaspoon	1 mL
½ teaspoon	2 mL
¾ teaspoon	4 mL
1 teaspoon	5 mL
1 tablespoon	15 mL
¼ cup	59 mL
⅓ cup	79 mL
½ cup	118 mL
⅔ cup	156 mL
¾ cup	177 mL
1 cup	235 mL
2 cups or 1 pint	475 mL
3 cups	700 mL
4 cups or 1 quart	1 L
½ gallon	2 L
1 gallon	4 L

OVEN TEMPERATURES

FAHRENHEIT (F)	CELSIUS (C) (APPROXIMATE)
250°F	120°C
300°F	150°C
325°F	165°C
350°F	180°C
375°F	190°C
400°F	200°C
425°F	220°C
450°F	230°C

WEIGHT EQUIVALENTS

US STANDARD	METRIC (APPROXIMATE)
½ ounce	15 g
1 ounce	30 g
2 ounces	60 g
4 ounces	115 g
8 ounces	225 g
12 ounces	340 g
16 ounces or 1 pound	455 g

REFERENCES

Abazarfard, Z., M. Salehi, and S. Keshavarzi. "The Effect of Almonds on Anthropometric Measurements and Lipid Profile in Overweight and Obese Females in a Weight Reduction Program: A Randomized Controlled Clinical Trial." *Journal of Research in Medical Sciences: the official journal of Isfahan University of Medical Sciences* 19, no. 5 (May 2014): 457–64. www.ncbi.nlm.nih .gov/pubmed/25097630.

Abugoch, James L. E. "Quinoa (Chenopodium quinoa Willd.): Composition, Chemistry, Nutritional, and Functional Properties." *Advances in Food and Nutrition Research* 58 (2009): 1–31. doi:10.1016/S1043-4526(09)58001-1. www.ncbi.nlm.nih.gov/pubmed/19878856.

Assunção, M. L., H. S. Ferreira, A. F. dos Santos, C. R. Cabral Jr., and T. M. Florêncio. "Effects of Dietary Coconut Oil on the Biochemical and Anthropometric Profiles of Women Presenting Abdominal Obesity." *Lipids* 44, no. 7 (July 2009): 593–601. doi:10.1007/s11745-009-3306-6. www.ncbi.nlm.nih.gov /pubmed/19437058.

Bailey, S. J., R. L. Varnham, F. J. DiMenna, B. C. Breese, L. J. Wylie, A. M. Jones. "Inorganic Nitrate Supplementation Improves Muscle Oxygenation, O_2 Uptake Kinetics, and Exercise Tolerance at High but Not Low Pedal Rates." *Journal of Applied Physiology (1985)* 118, no. 11 (June 2015): 1396–405. doi:10.1152 /japplphysiol.01141.2014. www.ncbi.nlm.nih.gov/pubmed/25858494.

BeefNutrition.org. "Many of America's Favorite Cuts Are Lean." PDF. Accessed July 21, 2016. www.beefitswhatsfordinner.com/CMDocs/BIWFD/FactSheets /Many_Of_Americas_Favorite_Cuts_Are_Lean.pdf.

CalorieKing. The Nutritional Information for a T-Bone Steak, Lean Only, Broiled. www.calorieking.com/foods/calories-in-beef-beef-t-bone-steak-lean-only -broiled_f-ZmlkPTYxMjI2.html.

Chang, H. P., M. L. Wang, M. H. Chan, Y. S. Chiu, Y. H. Chen. "Antiobesity Activities of Indole-3-Carbinol in High-Fat-Diet-Induced Obese Mice." *Nutrition* 27, no. 4 (April 2011): 463–70. doi:10.1016/j.nut.2010.09.006. www.ncbi.nlm.nih.gov /pubmed/21392705.

Chowdhury, E. A., J. D. Richardson, K. Tsintzas, D. Thompson, and J. A. Betts. "Carbohydrate-Rich Breakfast Attenuates Glycaemic, Insulinaemic and Ghrelin Response to Ad Libitum Lunch Relative to Morning Fasting in Lean Adults." *The British Journal of Nutrition* 114, no. 1 (July 2015): 98–107. doi:10.1017/S0007114515001506. Epub 2015 May 25. www.ncbi.nlm.nih.gov/pubmed/26004166.

Couturier, K., I. Hininger, L. Poulet, R. A. Anderson, A. M. Roussel, F. Canini, and C. Batandier. "Cinnamon Intake Alleviates the Combined Effects of Dietary-Induced Insulin Resistance and Acute Stress on Brain Mitochondria." *The Journal of Nutritional Biochemistry* 28 (February 2016): 183–90. doi:10.1016/j.jnutbio.2015.10.016. www.ncbi.nlm.nih.gov/pubmed/26878796.

Daley, C. A., A. Abbott, P.S. Doyle, G. A. Nader, and S. Larson. "A Review of Fatty Acid Profiles and Antioxidant Content in Grass-Fed and Grain-Fed Beef." *Nutrition Journal* 9, no. 10 (March 2010): doi:10.1186/1475-2891-9-10. www.ncbi.nlm.nih.gov/pubmed/20219103.

Davidson, M. H., L. D. Dugan, J. H. Burns, J. Bova, K. Story, and K. B. Drennan. "The Hypocholesterolemic Effects of Beta-Glucan in Oatmeal and Oat Bran. A Dose-Controlled Study." *Journal of the American Medical Association.* 265, no. 14 (April 1991): 1833–9. www.ncbi.nlm.nih.gov/pubmed/2005733.

De Santi, M., E. Carloni, L. Galluzzi, A. Diotallevi, S. Lucarini, M. Magnani, and G. Brandi. "Inhibition of Testosterone Aromatization by the Indole-3-carbinol Derivative CTet in CYP19A1-overexpressing MCF-7 Breast Cancer Cells." *Anticancer Agents in Medicinal Chemistry* 15, no. 7 (January 2015): 896–904. www.ncbi.nlm.nih.gov/pubmed/25612679.

Dullo, A. G., J. Seydoux, L. Girardier, P. Chantre, and J. Vancermander. "Green Tea and Thermogenesis: Interactions Between Catechin-Polyphenols, Caffeine and Sympathetic Activity." *The International Journal of Obesity* 24, no. 2 (February 2000): 252–258. www.ncbi.nlm.nih.gov/pubmed/10702779.

Freeland, J. H., and R. J. Cousins. "Zinc Content of Selected Foods." *The Journal of the American Dietetic Association* 68, no. 6 (June 1976): 526–9. www.ncbi.nlm.nih.gov/pubmed/1270715.

Granell, J. "Zinc and Copper Changes in Serum and Urine after Aerobic Endurance and Muscular Strength Exercise." *The Journal of Sports Medicine and Physical Fitness* 52, no. 2 (April 2014): 232–7. www.ncbi.nlm.nih.gov/pubmed/24509996.

Grimaldi, A. S., B. A. Parker, J. A. Capizzi, P. M. Clarkson, L. S. Pescatello, M. C. White, and P. D. Thompson. "25(OH) Vitamin D is Associated with Greater Muscle Strength in Healthy Men and Women." *Medicine and Science in Sports and Exercise* 45, no. 1 (January 2013): 157–62. doi:10.1249/MSS.0b013e31826c9a78. www.ncbi.nlm.nih.gov/pubmed/22895376.

Gutiérrez-Hellín, J, J. D. Coso. "Acute P-synephrine Ingestion Increases fat Oxidation Rate During Exercise." *British Journal of Clinical Pharmacology* 82, no. 2 (August 2016): 362–8. doi:10.1111/bcp.12952. www.ncbi.nlm.nih.gov/pubmed/27038225.

Haff, G. G., M. J. Lehmkuhl, L. B. McCoy, and M. H. Stone. "Carbohydrate Supplementation and Resistance Training." *The Journal of Strength and Conditioning Research* 17, no. 1 (February 2003): 187–96. www.ncbi.nlm.nih.gov/pubmed/12580676.

Harms-Ringdahl, Mats, Dag Jenssen, and Siamak Haghdoost. "Tomato Juice Intake Suppressed Serum Concentration of 8-oxodG after extensive Physical Activity." *Nutrition Journal* 11, no. 1 (May 2012): 29. doi:10.1186/1475-2891-11-29 www.ncbi.nlm.nih.gov/pubmed/22551119.

Hashemi, M., E. Khosravi, A. Ghannadi, M. Hashemipour, and R. Kelishadi. "Effect of the Peels of Two Citrus Fruits on Endothelium Function in Adolescents with Excess Weight: A Triple-Masked Random Trial." *Journal of Research in Medical Sciences: the official journal of Isfahan University of Medical Sciences* 20, no. 8 (August 2015): 721–6. doi:10.4103/1735-1995.168273. www.ncbi.nlm.nih.gov/pubmed/26664417.

Helms, E. R., A. A. Aragon, and P. J. Fitschen. "Evidence-Based Recommendations for Natural Bodybuilding Contest Preparation: Nutrition and Supplementation." *Journal of the International Society of Sports Nutrition* 11, no. 20 (2014): www.ncbi.nlm.nih.gov/pubmed/24864135.

Helms, E. R., C. Zinn, D. S. Rowlands, and S. R. Brown. "A Systematic Review of Dietary Protein During Caloric restriction in Resistance Trained Lean Athletes: A Case for Higher Intakes." *International Journal of Sport Nutrition and Exercise Metabolism* 24, no. 2 (April 2014):127–38. doi:10.1123/ijsnem. www.ncbi.nlm.nih.gov/pubmed/24092765.

Higdon, Jane, Victoria J. Drake, Giana Angelo, and Donald B. Jump. "Essential Fatty Acids." Linus Pauling Institute, Micronutrient Information Center. Oregon State University. Copyright 2003–2016 Linus Pauling Institute. Accessed July 21, 2016. http://lpi.oregonstate.edu/mic/other-nutrients/essential-fatty-acids.

Jenkins, D. J., C. W. Kendall, L. S. Augustin, S. Mitchell, S. Sahye-Pudaruth, S. Blanco Mejia, and L. Chiavaroli et al. "Effect of Legumes as Part of a Low Glycemic Index Diet on Glycemic Control and Cardiovascular Risk Factors in Type 2 Diabetes Mellitus: A Randomized Controlled Trial." *Archives of Internal Medicine* 172, no. 21 (November 2012):1653–60. www.ncbi.nlm.nih.gov/pubmed/23089999.

Jiang, T., X. Gao, C. Wu, F. Tian, Q. Lei, J. Bi, B. Xie, H. Y. Wang, S. Chen, and X. Wang. "Apple-Derived Pectin Modulates Gut Microbiota, Improves Gut Barrier Function, and Attenuates Metabolic Endotoxemia in Rats with Diet-Induced Obesity." *Nutrients* 8, no. 3 (February 2016): E126. doi:10.3390/nu8030126. www.ncbi.nlm.nih.gov/pubmed/26938554.

Jurgens, T. M., A. M. Whelan, L. Killian, S. Doucette, S. Kirk, and E. Foy. "Green Tea for Weight Loss and Weight Maintenance in Overweight or Obese Adults." *The Cochrane Database of Systematic Reviews* no. 12 (December 2012): CD008650. doi:10.1002/14651858.CD008650.pub2. www.ncbi.nlm.nih.gov/pubmed /23235664.

Karalus, M., and Z. Vickers. "Satiation and Satiety Sensations Produced by Eating Oatmeal vs. Oranges: A Comparison of Different Scales." *Appetite* 99 (April 2016): 168–76. doi:10.1016/j.appet.2016.01.012. www.ncbi.nlm.nih.gov /pubmed/26796421.

Katch, Frank I., and William D. McArdle. "Validity of Body Composition Prediction Equations for college Men and Women." *The American Journal of Clinical Nutrition* 28, no. 2 (February 1975): 105–109. http://ajcn.nutrition.org/content /28/2/105.extract.

Kelly, Mark P. "Resting Metabolic Rate: Best Ways to Measure It—And Raise It, Too" *The American Council of Exercise, Certified News*. October 2012. www.acefitness .org/certifiednewsarticle/2882/resting-metabolic-rate-best-ways-to-measure -it-and/.

Kelly, Mark B. Kerksick, Chad, Travis Harvey, Jeff Stout, Bill Campbell, Colin Wilborn, Richard Kreider, and Doug Kalman, et al. "International Society of Sports Nutrition position stand: Nutrient Timing." *Journal of the International Society of Sports Nutrition* 5, no. 17 (2008).

Kitakaze, T., N. Harada, H. Imagita, R. Yamaji. "β-Carotene Increases Muscle Mass and Hypertrophy in the Soleus Muscle in Mice." *Journal of Nutritional Science and Vitaminology* 61, no. 6 (2015): 481–7. doi:10.3177/jnsv.61.481. www.ncbi.nlm .nih.gov/pubmed/26875490.

Kunkel, S. D., M. Suneja, S. M. Ebert, K. S. Bongers, D. K. Fox, S. E. Malmberg, F. Alipour, R. K. Shields, C. M. Adams. "mRNA Expression Signatures of Human Skeletal Muscle Atrophy Identify a Natural Compound that Increases Muscle Mass." *Cell Metabolism* 13, no. 6 (June 2011): 627–38. doi:10.1016/j.cmet.2011.03.020. www.ncbi.nlm.nih.gov/pubmed/21641545.

Lam, C. K., Z. Zhang, H. Yu, S. Y. Tsang, Y. Huang, and Z. Y. Chen. "Apple Polyphenols Inhibit Plasma CETP Activity and Reduce the Ratio of Non-HDL to HDL Cholesterol." *Molecular Nutrition and Food Research* 52, no. 8 (August 2008): 950–8. doi:10.1002/mnfr.200700319. www.ncbi.nlm.nih.gov/pubmed/18496813.

Leidy, H. J., H. A. Hoertel, S. M. Douglas, K. A. Higgins, and R. S. Shafer. "A High-Protein Breakfast Prevents Body Fat Gain, through Reductions in Daily Intake and Hunger, in 'Breakfast Skipping' adolescents." *Obesity* 23, no. 9 (September 2015): 1761–4. doi:10.1002/oby.21185. www.ncbi.nlm.nih.gov/pubmed/26239831.

Linares, D. M., P. Ross, C. Stanton. "Beneficial Microbes: The Pharmacy in the Gut." *Bioengineered* 7, no. 1 (January 2016): 11–20. doi:10.1080/21655979.2015.1126015. www.ncbi.nlm.nih.gov/pubmed/26709457.

Lukyanenko, Y.O., J. J. Chen, J. C. Hutson. "Production of 25-hydroxycholesterol by Testicular Macrophages and Its Effects on Leydig Cells." *Biology of Reproduction* 64, no. 3 (March 2001): 790–6. www.ncbi.nlm.nih.gov/pubmed/11207193.

Maki, K. C., M. S. Reeves, M. Farmer, K. Yasunaga, N. Matsuo, Y. Katsuragi, and M. Komikado, et al. "Green Tea Catechin consumption Enhances Exercise-Induced Abdominal Fat Loss in Overweight and Obese Adults." *The Journal of Nutrition* 139, no. 2 (February 2009): 264–70. doi:10.3945/jn.108.098293. http://jn.nutrition.org/content/139/2/264.full.

Melanson, K., J. Gootman, A. Myrdal, G, Kline, and J. M. Rippe. "Weight Loss and Total Lipid Profile Changes in Overweight Women Consuming Beef or Chicken as the Primary Protein Source". *Nutrition* 19, no. 5 (May 2003): 409–414. www.ncbi.nlm.nih.gov/pubmed/12714091.

Miranda, J. M., M. Guarddon, A. Mondragon, B. L. Vasquez, C. A. Fente, A. Cepeda, and C. M. Franco. "Antimicrobial Resistance in Enterococcus Spp. Strains Isolated from Organic Chicken, Conventional Chicken, and Turkey Meat: A Comparative Survey." *The Journal of Food Protection* 70, no. 4 (April 2007): 1021–4. www.ncbi.nlm.nih.gov/pubmed/17477278.

Montelius, C., D. Erlandsson, E. Vitija, E. L. Stenblom, E. Egecioglu, and C. Erlanson-Albertsson. "Body Weight Loss, Reduced Urge for Palatable Food and Increased Release of GLP-1 through Daily Supplementation with Green-Plant Membranes for Three Months in Overweight Women." *Appetite* 81 (October 2014): 295–304. doi:10.1016/j.appet.2014.06.101. www.ncbi.nlm.nih.gov/pubmed/24993695.

Mori, T. A., V. Burke, I. B. Puddey, J. E. Shaw, L. J. Beilin. "Effect of Fish Diets and Weight Loss on Serum Leptin Concentration in Overweight, Treated-Hypertensive Subjects." *Journal of Hypertension* 22, no. 10 (October 2004): 1983–90. www.ncbi.nlm.nih.gov/pubmed/15361771.

Morris, M. C., D. A. Evans, C. C. Tangney, J. L. Bienias, and R. S. Wilson. "Fish Consumption and Cognitive Decline with Age in a Large Community Study." *Archives of Neurology* 62, no. 12 (December 2005): 1849–53. www.ncbi.nlm.nih.gov/pubmed/16216930.

Mozaffarian, Dariush, Tao Hao, Eric B. Rimm, Walter C. Willett, and Frank B. Hu. "Changes in Diet and Lifestyle and Long-Term Weight Gain in Women and Men." *New England Journal of Medicine* 364 (June 2011): 2392–2404. www.nejm.org/doi/full/10.1056/NEJMoa1014296.

Murphy, Karen J., Barbara Parker, Kathryn A. Dyer, Courtney R. Davis, Alison M. Coates, Jonathan D. Buckley, and Peter R. C. Howe. "A Comparison of Regular Consumption of Fresh Lean Pork, Beef and Chicken on Body Composition: A Randomized Cross-Over Trial." *Nutrients* 6, no. 2 (February 2014): 682–696. www.ncbi.nlm.nih.gov/pmc/articles/PMC3942727/.

National Heart, Lung, and Blood Institute, US Department of Health and Human Services. "Balance Food and Activity." Accessed July 21, 2016. www.nhlbi.nih.gov/health/educational/wecan/healthy-weight-basics/balance.htm.

Nieman, D. C., N. D. Gillitt, D. A. Henson, W. Sha, R. A. Shanely, A. M. Knab, L. Cialdella-Kam, and F. Jin. "Bananas as an Energy Source During Exercise: A Metabolomics Approach." *PLoS One* 7, no. 5 (May 2012): e37479. doi:10.1371/journal.pone.0037479. www.ncbi.nlm.nih.gov/pubmed/22616015.

Nimptsch, K., E. A. Platz, W. C. Willett, and E. Giovannucci. "Association Between Plasma 25-OH Vitamin D and Testosterone Levels in Men." *Clinical Endocrinology* 77, no. 1 (July 2012):106–12. doi:10.1111/j.1365-2265.2012.04332.x. www.ncbi.nlm.nih.gov/pubmed/22220644.

Ormsbee, M. J., C. W. Bach, and D. A. Baur. "Pre-Exercise Nutrition: The Role of Macronutrients, Modified Starches and Supplements on Metabolism and Endurance Performance." *Nutrients* 6, no. 5 (2014): 1782–1808. www.ncbi.nlm.nih.gov/pmc/articles/PMC4042570/.

Ostman, E., Y. Granfeldt, L. Persson, and I. Björck. "Vinegar Supplementation Lowers Glucose and Insulin Responses and Increases Satiety after a Bread Meal in Healthy Subjects." *European Journal of Clinical Nutrition* 59, no. 9 (September 2005): 983–8. www.ncbi.nlm.nih.gov/pubmed/16015276.

Paddon-Jones, Douglas, Eric Westman, Richard D. Mattes, Robert R. Wolfe, Arne Astrup, and Margriet Westerterp-Plantenga. "Protein, Weight Management, and Satiety." *The American Journal of Clinical Nutrition* 87, no. 5 (May 2008): 1558S–1561S http://ajcn.nutrition.org/content/87/5/1558S.long.

Pal, S., S. Radavelli-Bagatini. "Effects of Psyllium on Metabolic Syndrome Risk Factors." *Obesity Reviews: The Official Journal of the International Association for the Study of Obesity* 13, no. 11 (November 2012): 1034–47. doi:10.1111 /j.1467-789X.2012.01020.x. www.ncbi.nlm.nih.gov/pubmed/22863407.

Park, K. S. "Raspberry Ketone Increases Both Lipolysis and Fatty Acid Oxidation in 3T3-L1 Adipocytes." *Planta Medica* 76, no. 15 (October 2010): 1654–8. doi:10.1055/s-0030-1249860. www.ncbi.nlm.nih.gov/pubmed/20425690.

Phillips, S. "Dietary Protein for Athletes: From Requirements to Metabolic Advantage." *Applied Physiology, Nutrition, and Metabolism* 31, no. 6 (2006): 647–654. doi:10.1139/h06-035. www.ncbi.nlm.nih.gov/pubmed/17213878.

Phillips, S. M., and L. J. Van Loon. "Dietary Protein for Athletes: From Requirements to Optimum Adaptation." *Journal of Sports Sciences* 29, sup. 1 (2011): S29–38. doi:10.1080/02640414.2011.619204. www.ncbi.nlm.nih.gov /pubmed/22150425

Popkin, Barry M., Kristen E. D'Anci, Irwin H. Rosenberg. "Water, Hydration and Health." *Nutrition Reviews* 68, no. 8. (August 2010): 439–458. https://nutritionreviews.oxfordjournals.org/content/68/8/439.full.

Ruxton, C. H. S., S. C. Reed, M. J. A. Simpson, and K. J. Millington. "The Health Benefits of Omega-3 Polyunsaturated Fatty Acids: A Review of the Evidence." *The Journal of Human Nutrition and Dietetics* 17, no. 5 (October 2004): 449–459.

Ryberg, M., S. Sandberg, C. Mellberg, O. Stegle, B. Lindahl, C. Larsson, J. Hauksson, and T. Olsson. "A Palaeolithic-Type Diet Causes Strong Tissue-Specific Effects on Ectopic Fat Deposition in Obese Postmenopausal Women." *The Journal of Internal Medicine* 274, no. 1 (July 2013): 67–76. doi:10.1111/joim.12048. www.ncbi.nlm.nih.gov/pubmed/23414424.

Shishehbor, F., A. Mansoori, A. R. Sarkaki, M. T. Jalali, S. M. Latifi. "Apple Cider Vinegar Attenuates Lipid Profile in Normal and Diabetic Rats." *Pakistan Journal of Biological Sciences* 11, no. 23 (December 2008): 2634–8. www.ncbi.nlm.nih .gov/pubmed/19630216.

St. Jeor, Sachiko T., Barbara V. Howard, T. Elaine Prewitt, Vicki Bovee, Terry Bazzarre, and Robert H. Eckel. "AHA Science Advisory, Dietary Protein and Weight Reduction." *Circulation* 104, no. 15 (October 2001): 1869–1874 doi:10.1161/hc4001.096152. http://circ.ahajournals.org/content/104/15/1869.full.

Tekeleselassie, A. W., Y. M. Goh, M. A. Rajion, M. Motshakeri, and M. Ebrahimi. "A High-Fat Diet Enriched with Low Omega-6 to Omega-3 Fatty Acid Ratio Reduced Fat Cellularity and Plasma Leptin Concentration in Sprague-Dawley Rats." *The Scientific World Journal.* (October 2013): doi:10.1155/2013/757593. www.ncbi.nlm.nih.gov/pubmed/24294136.

Tong, H.B., Q. Wang, J. Lu, J. M. Zou, L. L. Chang, and S. Y. Fu. "Effect of Free-Range Days on a Local Chicken Breed: Growth Performance, Carcass Yield, Meat Quality, and Lymphoid Organ Index." *Poultry Science* 93, no. 8 (August 2014): 1883–9. doi:10.3382/ps.2013-03470. www.ncbi.nlm.nih.gov/pubmed/24931968.

Tremblay, A., H. Arguin, and S. Panahi. "Capsaicinoids: A Spicy Solution to the Management of Obesity?" *International Journal of Obesity* 2005. online publication, January 2016; doi:10.1038/ijo.2015.253. www.ncbi.nlm.nih.gov/pubmed/26686003.

Turocy, Paula Sammarone, Bernard F. DePalma, Craig A. Horswill, Kathleen M. Laquale, Thomas J. Martin, Arlette C. Perry, Marla J. Somova, and Alan C. Utter. "National Athletic Trainers' Association Position Statement: Safe Weight Loss and Maintenance Practices in Sport and Exercise." *The Journal of Athletic Training* 46, no. 3 (May–June 2011): 322–336. www.ncbi.nlm.nih.gov/pmc/articles/PMC3419563/.

Uemura, M., H. Yatsuya, E. H. Hilawe, Y. Li, C. Wang, C. Chiang, R. Otsuka, H. Toyoshima, K. Tamakoshi, and A. Aoyama. "Breakfast Skipping Is Positively Associated with Incidence of Type 2 Diabetes Mellitus: Evidence from the Aichi Workers' Cohort Study." *The Journal of Epidemiology/ Japan Epidemiological Association* 25, no. 5 (2015): 351–8. doi:10.2188/jea.JE20140109. www.ncbi.nlm.nih.gov/pubmed/25787236.

United States Department of Agriculture. "Why Is It Important to Eat Vegetables?" Accessed July 21, 2016. www.choosemyplate.gov/vegetables-nutrients-health.

US Department of Agriculture, Agricultural Research Service. USDA National Nutrient Database for Standard Reference, Release 26. 2014. http://ndb.nal.usda.gov/.

Vanhatalo, A., A. M. Jones, J. R. Blackwell, P. G. Winyard, and J. Fulford. "Dietary Nitrate Accelerates Postexercise Muscle Metabolic Recovery and O2 Delivery in Hypoxia." *Journal of Applied Physiology* 117, no. 12 (December 2014): 1460–70. doi:10.1152/japplphysiol.00096.2014. www.ncbi.nlm.nih.gov /pubmed/25301896.

Westerterp-Plantenga, M. S., A. Sneets, and M. P. Lejeune. "Sensory and Gastrointestinal Satiety Effects of Capsaicin on Food Intake." *International Journal of Obesity* 29, no. 6 (June 2005): 682–8 www.ncbi.nlm.nih.gov /pubmed/26686003.

Witard, O. C., S. L. Wardle, L. S. Macnaughton, A. B. Hodgson, and K. D. Tipton. "Protein Considerations for Optimising Skeletal Muscle Mass in Healthy Young and Older Adults." *Nutrients* 8, no. 4 (March 2016): E181. doi:10.3390/nu8040181. www.ncbi.nlm.nih.gov/pubmed/27023595.

Witbracht, M., N. L. Keim, S. Forester, A. Widaman, and K. Laugero. "Female Breakfast Skippers Display a Disrupted Cortisol Rhythm and Elevated Blood Pressure." *Physiology and Behavior* 140 (March 2015): 215–21. doi:10.1016 /j.physbeh.2014.12.044. www.ncbi.nlm.nih.gov/pubmed/25545767.

Wylie, L. J., J. Kelly, S. J. Bailey, J. R. Blackwell, P. F. Skiba, P. G. Winyard, A. E. Jeukendrup, A. Vanhatalo, and A. M. Jones. "Beetroot Juice and Exercise: Pharmacodynamic and Dose-Response Relationships." *The Journal of Applied Physiology* 115, no. 3 (August 2013): 325–36. doi:10.1152 /japplphysiol.00372.2013. www.ncbi.nlm.nih.gov/pubmed/23640589.

Yoneshiro, T., A. Aita, Y. Kawai, T. Iwanaga, and Saito M. "Nonpungent Capsaicin Analogs (Capsinoids) Increase Energy Expenditure Through the Activation of Brown Adipose Tissue in Humans." *The American Journal of Clinical Nutrition* 95, no. 4 (April 2012): 845–50. doi:10.3945/ajcn.111.018606. www.ncbi.nlm.nih.gov /pubmed/22378725.

ABOUT THE AUTHOR

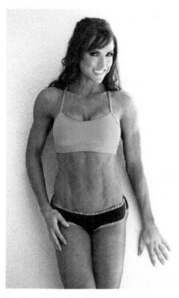

KENDALL LOU SCHMIDT brings a broad range of sport and educational experience to her personal training. A graduate of UC Davis, Kendall received a Bachelor's Degree in Biological Sciences with an emphasis in Neurobiology, Physiology and Behavior. For over a decade, she has been working in fitness and wellness as a personal trainer, group fitness instructor, coach, motivational & educational public speaker, presenter and examiner for the Aerobics and Fitness Association of America and, most recently, as the Northern California Instructor Coordinator for the Silver Sneakers Fitness Program.

Kendall has also led the UC Davis Football, Basketball, Gymnastics, and Women's Swim Team through preseason conditioning. She has enjoyed training triathletes, instructing swim lessons, teaching diverse group fitness classes and training clients of all fitness levels, ages, and backgrounds. Kendall is skilled in helping clients develop programs that complement their busy lifestyles. With her training, she continues to inspire and engage, breaking through fitness plateaus and keeping her clients motivated.

Kendall has competed in dozens of NPC Bikini competitions on both a regional and national level. She has been honored as a contributing author, sponsored athlete, and spokesmodel. In 2014, she was selected as one of five female finalists in the Bodybuilding.com BodySpace Spokesmodel Search. She lives in Sacramento, California.

RECIPE INDEX

INDEX

CPSIA information can be obtained
at www.ICGtesting.com
Printed in the USA
LVOW05s0152091216

516067LV00001BA/1/P